2nd Edition

The Dragonfly Approach

of Pediatric Occupational Therapy

A practical guide of what to do after your child's diagnosis.

By: Sharon Y. Mandeville-Edlin, OTR/L

Praise for The Dragonfly Approach

"This book has fresh ideas and good reminders of what is important at the end of the day which is happiness and the well-being of the child and family! This book is written with open-minded suggestions for parents and professionals."

–Kirsten (a mother of a child with special needs)

"The easy writing style gave me great insight into so many aspects of my life and the life of my children. This book will help EVERYONE understand children and even adults better."

–Lisa (a mother of a child with special needs)

"Excellent straight to the meat book. It is very easy to read and one you don't want to put down once you start! It feels like she is talking to you."

–Tami (a mother of a child with special needs)

Disclaimer

Every effort has been made to ensure the accuracy of the content in this book. The author assumes no liability for any inaccuracy or incompleteness, as it was not done on purpose. If you have any additional or helpful information, I'd love for you to relay it to me for I am very open-minded and love learning.

The information provided in the book is designed to provide helpful, down-to-earth, written in layman's terms with a heavy sprinkle of 27 years of being an Occupational Therapist (OT). The way in which I do these things is known as 'The Dragonfly Approach.' This book is not meant to diagnose as we OTs aren't authorized to do so. For diagnosis of any medical issue, consult your physician and show him/her this book, it could help lead you in the right direction. If your child is already receiving occupational therapy or physical therapy or speech therapy, I urge you to ask them about the information in this book.

I am not responsible for any specific health or allergy needs that may require medical supervision and I'm also not liable for any damage or negative consequences from any treatment, action, application, or preparation to any person reading this

book. The references that I provided are for informational purposes only and do not constitute endorsements of any websites or other sources.

This book is dedicated to all parents everywhere

Table of Contents

What is a Pediatric Occupational Therapist?

The abbreviation I will use throughout this book is "OT"

Pediatric Occupational Therapists utilize therapeutic play to address areas of delayed development. These areas include fine-motor skills such as buttoning, holding a pencil properly, and handwriting; gross-motor skills such as kicking a ball, climbing, and hopping on one leg, and general coordinated movements used to play on the playground, for example; visual perceptual and motor skills such as copying from the whiteboard or putting together a puzzle; general visual skills such as tracking issues and visual convergence; sensory integration, which is the ability to organize the information we receive from all 7 senses in a functional way; core strength; brain-body remapping/connection; retained neonatal reflexes; timing, sequencing, and attention; and for my unique practice, diet, which is of utmost importance. I help build confidence and provide vital education and home exercise programs for both my OT kids and their families.

I'm also a shoulder to cry on, a friend, a sounding board, a best friend, a cowgirl, a cashier, a magic princess, a robot, a pretend sister, a glittery unicorn, a stormtrooper, and many other roles that my OT kids assign me each week in therapy. I have the greatest job in the world!

Why I Can Write This Book with Earned Authority

Hey there, and welcome to a book that might certainly change you and your child's life. I say 'special needs' in the title but I think the information that I will give you throughout this book can apply to any child today. Especially for a sibling of a special needs child. That is why I added that last part in the title because every child (and I believe adults as well) can benefit from what I am going to talk to you about. The reason I say any child, is because the things that you are going to learn, I used on my own two children, and neither of them would be considered special needs by today's standards. However, each time I see a new 'OT kid,' I always tell them my beginning story as a child myself, and then I tell them about my own kids, and I'll tell you straight up, this sets the perfect trust foundation with the kids I work with, it really does. They feel they are not alone and not so far removed from everyone else because "Ms. Sharon has been there and gets me."

Let me back up and explain why I have been there and why I can write this book with utter 'been-there-done-that' confidence . . .

I was born 100 years ago in Springfield, Illinois, yes, the Land of Lincoln. Okay, not 100 years ago but in 1971. I was born to a father of 23 years old and a mother who had just turned 20 a few weeks before my birth. She was a child herself but a darn good mother, I can assure you. We were not a wealthy family by any means but my father was a very hard worker and my mom did plenty to make money from home while taking care of us such as having a daycare at her house, selling homemade candy at the holiday's, breeding and selling dachshund puppies, and a million other things to contribute to our middle-income household.

I am the eldest of two sisters who were born only 15 months apart. Back then, you didn't hear terms like gluten, MSG, GMO'S, autism, genetic disorders, hormones in your meat, etc., etc. We were just simple folk living through the '70s.

In addition to being allergic to cow's milk as a baby (I will touch a lot on why I do not recommend cow's milk in any child's diet later on this the book, so stay tuned), resulting in sleeping for only 45 minutes at a time, I also had horrible asthma, undiagnosed ADHD, dyslexia, and sensory integration issues. The reason I say undiagnosed is that back then, folks just thought hyperactive insane looking children were just 'busy' and dyslexia sounded like someone was cussing at you in another language. There was very little testing for issues back in the '70s and no one was questioning what was in those vaccinations they were making everyone get. Plus, my mom tells me that if a kid did get plagued with a diagnosis of ADHD, they'd throw pills at the kid thus rendering them a zombie. That bothered my mom and she was always concerned about the side effects of medication on the human body.

I went to a Catholic school at the time and <u>some</u> of the nuns were quite interesting, I can tell you that. In this particular school, if you didn't fit 'the mold' you were treated differently essentially as all children just want to 'belong.' Well, I didn't fit the mold, and here's why.

I'd say I was in the first or second grade when this little incident happened involving math class. For some freaking ridiculous reason, that I did not understand at the time, our teacher decided that we would learn a part of math using beans. Yes, beans. I have no idea why so don't even ask. So, if I remember right, we were learning to count by 5's and 10's and had to group our beans in these two units/groups to get whatever answer the teacher was looking for. My mom tells me that I would already know the answer without using the stupid beans but that the teacher wouldn't give me credit because I wouldn't use my beans. I thought it was ridiculous!

One day, I decided that I would just eat my beans therefore never having to use the little suckers again, well, in Catholic school, when you eat the beans, you get sent to special education (special ed) jail, evidently, and that's where I remained for 3 years. Now, eventually, special ed did help me because I ended up falling behind in reading and math, but initially, it was just jail for being a cannibal bean-eating murderer.

Once there, I quickly learned that it was not my cup of tea as I was the only girl in the 'jail' and the nun that ran special ed had some sort of fantasy that I was the daughter she never had and had finally discovered. It freaked me the heck out!

I struggled with reading and math, especially math, and math is still a challenge for me today, praise the Lord for calculators and my math-savvy children, who help their mom out a lot in this area.

I ended up being one of those kids that you hear about 'falling through the cracks' in a supposedly well put together school system because the special ed nun was so enamored by my daughterly-like presence, she kept me, prisoner, for 3 years, even though it was clear it was time for me to launch from special ed earlier than that. Cue, my warrior mother . . .

My mom is a Mama Bear Warrior and you don't mess with her 'Shari," as I was called 100 years ago. Once she figured out that I was doing pretty well and that I was being held prisoner by the crazy (well-intentioned) nun of special ed, she lost it and bailed me out, finally.

However, the stigma of not only being in special ed but also the only girl in there stuck with me for a long long time. Feeling different felt like I had my shirt and pants on backward or my shoes on the wrong feet, know what I mean? It just felt weird and uneasy in my heart, mind, and confidence.

So, this started the thought process that I was not capable of great things because there was something 'wrong' with me.

My mom knew that my 'hyperactivity' needed to be tamed so I was stuck into every sport she could find to wear me the heck out and out of all of them, softball stuck and I ended up being a catcher for 13 years. This organized sport plus the fast pace of being a catcher really helped me with my ADHD. I was also oddly strong and had Popeye forearms because of the steroids I was on for my asthma. No one messed with me during my softball years, I can assure you.

So, I knew or presumed I knew because of special ed, that I sucked at school but I was great at sports and that sports made my body and mind feel really good. Sports kept my self-esteem from plummeting and to some extent, helped me learn to focus.

Keep this in mind parents if you have an athletic child, go for it with the sports, but don't force athletics on a kid that hates it or isn't very good at it. That's like forcing you to eat liver and onions because it's 'good for you,' which now research has shown that eating liver is very bad for you. Don't do that to your kids, find something else like karate, yoga, archery, horseback riding, swimming, chess club, etc. You can't force a square into a circle, you will get resistance and grief, don't do it, not to mention when that kid of yours isn't as good as the rest of the kids, it will just add to the spiral downward!

Now, the discovery that I actually had dyslexia came when I began working as an OT for a dyslexia school in my late 30's, which was eye-opening for me, as I didn't know that's what was going on. It was probably the main reason for my trouble with math and reading, but you know what? I figured it out. The mind and body have an enormous capacity for adaptation, and your kids will too with just a bit of guidance from folks like me who have been there and just so happen to be a seasoned OT.

*****

A major event happened to me right after I turned 13 years old and it set my world on two wheels going around a curve traveling entirely too fast in the rain on a dark and stormy night.

My dad made the decision to quit his job because it had been sold to a foreign country. This meant that the company would be moving out of the country so my dad had to find himself a new job, which just so happened to be located in the South.

My first question was, "Um, hey dad. Do the folks down South have running water and electricity," as I was looking for any excuse to not have to move. Moving meant I'd have to leave my friends and wouldn't be playing volleyball on the team I had made.

So, just when I had finally launched from special ed, found a new best friend, and started to be sweet on a kid named Pete, we were given this devastating news about moving down South and I was petrified. I had finally adapted to my surroundings and knew what to expect on most days and now, I felt like I was starting over.

The first thing on my mind was, "Will I be put back into special ed because it was a new school, and would some crazy nun get ahold of me?" Well, my mom couldn't get all three of us into the Catholic school, praise

God, so we got the shocking surprise of going to a public school.

If the southern drawl wasn't enough, the gobs of make-up, scantily dressed girls (my perception because I was used to a most comfortable- not! -polyester uniform), rough-looking guys, and so many people in one place I'm not quite sure how kids didn't flip out because I certainly was. I was very much questioning my parent's sketchy decision to move to this insane place called the South.

Well, much to my surprise, because I went to a private school and it was a bit tougher, I actually did well throughout middle school but was not at all comfortable with all the make-up, clothing, and getting asked on the first day of school, "Will you go with me," which I had no idea what that meant so I asked the little dude where he wanted to go exactly because clearly he was a stranger and I just don't go off with anyone. My response just added to the 'appeal' screaming off of his little person, as he laughed so hard, I feared he'd pee himself, the little weirdo. Plus, I also didn't get the question, "Who ya for," to which I would reply, "Well, I'm for Jesus, who you for?" I'd get a laugh out of that as well but what I didn't realize is 'who ya for' meant were you for Alabama or Auburn. I discovered early on that this football stuff was serious business down here.

Good grades came to a screeching halt when I entered high school.

For some reason, the raging hormones in my body made concentration and focus next to impossible. I was flipping numbers, words, and letters more than I had in the past and kept having to go over and over my work, which was so infuriating.

My parents and sisters began to question if I was going to be able to cut it at college or would I be one of those failure to launch situations. That got to me, it really did.

*****

I can say with absolute honesty that high school was a living hell. In addition to below-average (math) to average grades, poor concentration, hormones, worsening dyslexia, and 10,000 bodies all in one place trying to get to opposites ends of the building in different directions, my social life took off and many ill decisions were made along the way. No, I didn't end up a teen pregnant chick or do drugs but I did get my first boyfriend who wanted to French kiss me on our second date and I had never kissed anyone before. Having a boyfriend became yet another distraction to my already distracted self.

I had just put a fresh piece of gum in my mouth and this is what I said in response to his suggestion to kiss, "Oh well, no I can't, I just put a new piece of gum in my mouth. I don't want to have to take it out. Sorry, maybe next time."

Yes, that is what I said and I'll bet you a dime to a dollar you can take a wild guess at what his face looked like, I won't even tell you, I'll leave it up to you. Lol!

To describe high school vaguely as a living hell is a bit of a cop-out on my part because I want you to understand what having 'issues' like mine looks and feels like, thus understanding your own kids a bit better.

On the first day of high school, I nearly threw up several times because of the fear of all the newness and the stories about the Seniors doing horrid things to freshmen. In addition to being what I called 'slightly claustrophobic,' I had something else going on with me that I knew was different from most people, like when I got into a crowd, I would literally feel like I was going to scream and melt away because of all the noise, the closeness, the smells, the body heat, etc. Now that we are on the subject, I also hated tags in my clothes, got car sick all of the time if I sat in the back seat, and could not spin or I'd vomit. Later on, I also discovered I got air sickness as well when I went on my first flight at 21 years old. The dude next to me was not a happy camper as I hurled several times in my assigned bag and then had to borrow his. Lol, poor fella.

I had no idea that in addition to ADHD and dyslexia, I'd discover that I had this other nugget of 'different-ness' called sensory processing disorder or SPD. At the time, I also had several retained reflexes that were the foundation of my SPD, but I'll get to that later.

You are now starting to see why I can and had to write this book because I have lived these issues all of my life and that is why I 'get' a lot of these OT kids I see. It doesn't go away without certain treatments and in some cases can get worse.

So, back to high school . . .

Every day was hard because of all of the bodies always around pressing the life out of me as I tried to make it to class on time. The noise was unbearable sometimes in between classes in the halls and it made me so stinkin' stabby that I'm pretty sure most people thought it was 'my time of the month' like every day.

It was pure overstimulation from too many people in one place plus the stress of getting to class on time. When my Sophomore year came around, my anger and frustration from having untreated ADHD, dyslexia, and my undiagnosed SPD/retained reflexes other thingy I didn't know I had, took their toll in the form of some very bad depression. Keep this in mind, parents, during those high school years with your kids. This is what might be going on and it is very real for them as it was for me.

I hated myself, I hated my room, I doubted there was a God, I hated my sisters, I hated what my mom got me for Christmas, and on and on. It was very bad!

And as the years finally brought me to my Senior year, I could not wait to bust out of that insane overcrowded asylum because anything was better than this.

****

Now let me just tell you a thing or two about that stinkin' freakin' satanic evil ACT. This test in no way accurately measures the mental intelligence, diligence, or the emotional intelligence of a person, no way Jose. In quoting the two dudes from the book called "The EQ Edge: Emotional Intelligence and Your Success" by Steven J. Stein, PH. D and Howard E. Book, MD:

"It is scarcely a revelation that not everyone's talents fit the school system's rather restrictive model for measuring achievement. History is full of brilliant, successful men and women who failed miserably or underachieved in the classroom, and whose teachers and guidance counselors relegated them to life on the margin. But despite this convincing body of evidence about emotional intelligence, society persisted in believing that success in school equals success in life or, at the very least, in the workplace."

This book has successfully overturned the very idea that the ACT measures the endless possibilities of a person and I'd like to say, "It's about dang time!"

Here is how this applied to me, and probably many of your children, as you sit and wring your hands worrying about their future. Deep breaths, people. It's going to be okay.

The highest score I could get on the ACT was a freaking 17; yes, you read that right, a 17. Here's why . . . I took the satanic evil test 3 times and each time they had this same lady in dang stiletto heels who would walk up and down the aisle and her heels made this 'clickity clickity clickity' sound and how do you think that translates to a person with ADHD. NOT WELL, people, I can assure you. I'm not sure why someone would wear these types of heels anyway, as I was pretty sure we weren't at a pole dancing class. Who the heck dresses like that for the satanic evil ACT student-monitoring job anyway?

Each time stiletto lady clicked by me, it would literally cause me to tear my eyes and my attention away from the task at hand- we can't help ourselves- to watch her walk by, not her actually, but her dang shoes. It's kind of like telling us to perpetually hold our breath, we can't, we just can't.

So, I graduate somehow with a sad 17 on the ACT and about a 2.5 GPA. Someone looking at me on paper would shake their head and pass me up at this point, but it was not at all what I was capable of.

Cue the sisters and parents . . .

"You have got to show more effort because we are not supporting you. You need to work hard in college; this is real life, Sharon. No more messing around."

"You're going to live with 'mommy' and 'daddy' forever. How does that make you feel?"

Thanks, fam, I appreciate it, but really, they had no idea what I'd end up being capable of and although these words stung, they helped in ways I would have never dreamed of.

P.S. I have an awesome family but they were all trying to put the scare into me to do better than I had been. For that, I love them.

****

Ah, good ole college, real-life, holy cow, this is really happening, how in the heck am I going to do this?

Because my ACT and GPA were so low, I was on probation the first semester of school. Oh, that just sounds peachy but at least they let me in. They being UAH, which was in town because my parents wanted to make sure I could cut it and I didn't blame them, I often doubted it myself.

My goal was to end up at UAB so I could get my Occupational Therapy degree but the competition to do this was incredibly fierce so I had to kick my butt into gear and guess what, I did! Yep, I found it in me and I never lost it once that momentum started going in the direction of something I felt passionate about.

At the end of the first semester at UAH, my 'probation officer' asked me how in the world I managed straight A's when my high school grades and unsavory ACT score showed a different picture. If I had known then what I know now, I would have climbed up on his too big for his office desk and told him straight up that numbers and grades do not define a person and that the system they have put together does not celebrate people who have in them more than you judgy counselors and teachers give us credit for. It was at that moment when he asked me how I managed straight A's that I thought, "You know what, I got this. I'm going to challenge myself to see if I can get straight A's all the way through. It's going to be hard as heck, but I will find a way to make this happen."

And in that defining moment, I pulled something out of me that looked a lot like determination, a lot like 'failure is not an option,' and a whole different perspective on how I wanted my future life to look like.

The year I applied to OT school with a 4.0, yes, a 4.0, 368 people had applied for 30 slots. I was terrified and confident all at the same time. Terrified of my competition but confidant that my grades, my attitude, my determination, and all of the volunteer work I had done at various facilities would pay off and, in the end, it did. By the Grace of God and my hard work, it did.

****

My dream of getting into OT school had come true and as I looked back on my life before, I was a bit disappointed I couldn't get it together then because I knew I had disappointed my parents. I think it all worked out the way it was supposed to because the way I figured it, if I had gotten this momentum in high school, it may have petered out by the time I got to college so I thought, "Everything happens for a reason, Sharon."

OT school was some of the hardest stuff I had ever had to learn and study and for some reason, there was an incredible sense of competition to see who could get the best grades, which became very motivating for me. Also, I had finally figured out what worked for me as far as study habits go as I didn't have any in high school. Nothing could be on the walls. Nothing on my desk other than what I was studying, shades closed on the window, no music, and no ticking or clicking sounds of any kind.

Now my roommate was the exact opposite of me. She had to have music and any other noise possible, TV, radio, etc. while she studied. She could actually sit by the pool at our apartment complex and study. This floored me.

If she had her music a bit too loud or she had finished studying and had folks over, I'd have to retreat into my walk-in closet with all of the sound muffling clothing, shut the door, and then I could keep studying.

Yes, this was my life at college, silence and absolutely no distraction but I figured it out, and that's what matters.

So, long story short, I kicked butt in OT school and left with a 4.0 and a Bachelor's degree. I was bursting with pride and my parents were amazed at what I was capable of for they did not see this early on. Failure was not an option anymore!

Now, the OT certification test was another story. I studied everything I could think of but those memories of that evil ACT kept coming back to haunt me. I would have nightmares about it fearing I'd fail the certification exam and all my hard work would be for nothing.

Well, a couple of good things happened. For one, there was carpeting in the testing room so no clickity heel sounds would distract me and, two, I was more prepared than I realized. All of the self-discovery I had done over the last 4 ½ years about myself paid off and I passed the certification exam without issue. Thank you, sweet baby Jesus.

****

After OT school, I wasn't quite sure what I wanted to specialize in but I did know that kids freaked me the heck out so I would definitely not go that route. You may be sitting there thinking, "What? Don't you work with kids now?"

I had never really been around little kids other than my freakish sisters, they really aren't freakish, but they did annoy the stew out of me when we were kids so to me, all kids were crazy. I was also worried that I'd break children somehow, not that I would do this on purpose, this was just my weird mindset. So, given that, I chose to work with adults after graduation.

Something happened to me while I was in OT school, it was called 'directed passion,' something I had never experienced before. Passion eluded me before because of all the sadness in myself and my heart that I was dealing with and my lost and feeling 'different' attitude.

I ended up at an inpatient rehabilitation center complete with a therapeutic pool. Cue the aquatic therapy passion . . .

I went nuts getting every class and certification under my belt for aquatic therapy. I also got crazy about stroke and head injury folks and quickly racked up more specialties and certifications. I sat on a board at some point for coming up with new ideas and treatment for these folks and eventually found myself in Atlanta on occasion, working in a cooperative effort with the spinal cord injury specialty center. Thus, becoming passionate about spinal cord injured patients as well.

I had released something in my person that I had never known before and would read anything I could get my hands on to be better at helping folks have the best quality of life possible. Directed passion is a very good thing, but it has to come from within, no one can give it to you. I was passionate all over the place at this point.

Cue the meeting of my future husband who would later be my ex.

****

Everything happens for a reason, they say. I have a bone to pick with 'they' I'm telling you right now.

In OT school I had to do several internships, some of them were short and some of them were long. One of my long ones took place in Grand Junction, Colorado arranged by me with permission from my OT school. I was pumped because I had always wanted to live in Colorado here's why . . .

From the time I was a tiny baby child, my parents took us there every summer for vacation. I inevitably fell in love with Colorado and swore that this incredibly gorgeous place would be where I'd end up living for the rest of my days. Ha, life has a way of doing its own thing . . .

After a fabulous internship, I was offered a job but the pay would make me poor and living on the streets in a box so I told my 'future' boss that I'd head back South to work at a job I was offered that paid a lot more, I'd save, and then I'd be back in a year.

Alas, in that year of saving and planning to get back out West, I met my future husband and lived the next challenging 16 years with him but when you are Catholic, you grin and bear it, and yes, a year to the day I got the call to work at that job I'd been offered in my sweet Colorado and it nearly killed me to turn it down.

Those 16 years were rough but it did give me my two blessings that would shape my future as a Pediatric Occupational Therapist, therefore, uncovering my true purpose on this Earth.

Up to this point, I had worked with geriatrics and adults in OT. I loved it, I was good at it, and I thought that's what I was supposed to be doing, until...

From the moment my son popped out, I was amazed, mesmerized, and floored by this little tiny person that had come out of my body. I had grown a whole person with and in my body. That was profound, and he sparked something in me I didn't think would ever be there . . . the love of pediatrics.

****

Why didn't I start here to begin with? This is what I asked myself as I watched my son each day barf, burp, cry, roll over, fart, sit up, crawl, stand up, walk, and all of the other things they do. I became obsessed with learning anything and everything I could about babies from an OT standpoint.

In the meantime, I was getting restless staying at home all day with my lovely son, and my then-husband was getting a bit nervous about money so I ended up working in the school systems part-time and again, so began another passion, being the best pediatric OT around.

I wanted to know EVERYTHING there was to know so I could help these kids in any way that I could. Again, I took every class, got every certification, and did a ton of self-study so I could help these kids soar. It also dawned on me at this time that I knew a heck of a lot more personally than a lot of my OT colleagues because I had lived some of these kid's struggles all my life.

After my daughter was born, I realized that I was so unbelievably limited in the school systems to give these kids what they truly needed because you can't work in a hallway or a janitor's closet and provide proper OT. Thus, my current practice was born.

Cue Daisy the Dragonfly, the little cute dragonfly on the front of this book, she's my logo and my inspiration in addition to my two children…

****

With extreme apprehension for fear of failure, I started my own private OT practice in the year 1999 because I was determined to treat these kids in a way that was right, good, and successful. I was also losing tons of sleep from the guilt I felt working in the school systems because I was not giving the kids my full capacity, that and the limited resources afforded to me at each school. I mean let's face it; you can only pack mule so much OT equipment into each school without breaking your back.

My clinic is the best thing that has happened to my passion and me since the birth of my two inspirational children. It is set up in my home in my converted two-car garage and I will have to say that I have never had a kid that didn't love coming to a 'home.' Once there, none of them want to leave, which is an incredible honor for me. The OT kids have also asked me if they can have sleepovers at my clinic and just the other day one of them asked if they could have their birthday party at my clinic. Oh, my heart just bursts in these moments.

Because of my practice, I have been able to raise my children on my own terms and along the way, I actually had to do OT treatment with each of them, here's what I mean.

My son was a bit sensitive to wind and water on his face. This baffled me until I found out that my then-husband would flip out while giving him a bath when the water got on his face and was quick to wipe it off with a washcloth offering a new way of thinking for my son to become more sensitive to things that had to do with his face. He probably had the platform for it but his dad became the launching mechanism as well as giving a heads up to my son's Reticular Activating System (RAS).

In a nutshell, this system is the set of connected nuclei in the brain that controls the sleep/wake cycle as well as what goes noticed or unnoticed by your system more or less.

So, I broke this pattern in two ways, giving the baths myself and starting the brushing and joint compression program with my son to desensitize his sensitivity. He also has ADHD and sensory processing issues with underlying retained reflexes. More on that later.

My daughter, on the other hand, had overall gross motor coordination delay and was falling so much I feared the wrath of DHR would be at my doorstep from all the bruises. She was also crazy impulsive and would often get hurt and had one messed up proprioceptive system (the system in the joints and muscle bellies that lets you know how hard or soft to hold an egg, for example) as she would hold the frogs she caught way too tight . . . you can figure out that outcome I'm sure. RIP, little froggie. She was put on an OT program as well and with time, I fixed her right up too.

Yes, in addition to all of my issues of ADHD, dyslexia, and sensory processing disorder/retained reflexes, I thought I had passed the ADHD and SPD to my kids but later on, I would find some jaw-dropping information from a man named Anthony William/Spirit aka The Medical Medium.

The fact that my own kids' struggle, allows me to feel another layer of what it must be like to be a parent of a kid with 'special needs.' Again, given today's standards being a bit more severe when you say 'special needs,' my kids are mild, I guess, and well heck, I guess I'm a mild special needs person too now that I think about it, and I have had trials as you have read.

So, here I am, I have issues of my own and have felt them all of my life (still do), I am an OT and own a pediatric clinic seeing kids with special needs every day, and my kids had/have issues. I consider myself the trifecta of understanding. Wouldn't you agree?

These are the reasons I can write this book and give you all of the knowledge I have absorbed over the last 27 years of being an OT.

From here, I will talk about observation, testing, the right way to treat your child, diet, and a lot more. Go get your popcorn and soft drink, folks, this just got real.

Primitive Reflexes Part 1

A lot of folks think of the knee-jerk reaction when they hear the word 'reflex.' The knee-jerk reaction is when your doctor clobbers your knee with his miniature evil hammer and your leg involuntarily kicks out and yes, that is a reflex but there are A LOT more. There are actually 70 known primary reflexes but for our purposes, I am referring to the ones that most affect children from the ages of 8 months to 18 months old. However, many adults still have retained reflexes, like me, my mom, and my husband, for example, which I will explain later.

Retained primitive reflexes, as I see it, are affecting probably 50%+ of the general population of kids, my opinion and not researched, just years and years of being around people and children and again, this is the layman/professional book of knowledge. I could throw big huge 're-searchy' words at you but really, what good would that do? You'd put the book down or better yet, get on Amazon and start the return process, so no, that's not how I am rolling here. Let's keep it simple but awesome.

Before I go on to explain these primitive reflexes, I must address the folks out there that say that retained reflexes don't exist. Obviously, they have not worked with human people or followed the testing processes involved in discovering them. Apparently, they live their lives in perfect harmony with their bodies and their bodies have never done anything unusual. You people are nuts and need to do some research and test and work with 'human' people. I can tell you with absolute certainty that these retained reflexes do exist and I have seen them in my mom, husband (the man I had the privilege of marrying after my failed 16-year marriage to my first husband), my own kids, myself, and many many of my OT kids. I have tested and treated them and have had amazing reports/gains from not only my OT kids but for myself, my own kids, and my husband. Experience is my guide and it should be yours too.

****

Primitive reflexes are found in the brain stem, which is the oldest part of our brain. It's the roots, if you will, of where everything essentially starts. The brain stem is responsible for breathing, swallowing, heart rate, blood pressure, and whether one is awake or sleeping (that Reticular Activating System I spoke of earlier.) It also controls the messages between our brain and our body.

I once saw a picture of a brain and it explained that the brain essentially develops from the brain stem up so as you get to the tip of the brain, where your halo would be, that's where the much more complex things happen such as language, vision, etc.

An aside here…I have seen many a therapist treat from the top of the brain down. You may ask, "What does this strange crazy OT mean?" Well, if a child is having trouble with handwriting, for example, and you keep throwing fine-motor exercises at them as well as hours of practicing handwriting and you don't seem to be making any progress with their handwriting, then you've started at the wrong end of the brain essentially. You've got to go back to that brain stem, the roots of the brain, and figure out what's going down there.

I'd equate what I'm talking about in practical terms to sitting in front of an <u>unlit</u> campfire with your marshmallow on a stick holding it over the 'non-fire' to make those awesome s'mores you love. Um, well, what's wrong with this picture? Is your marshmallow going to cook without a fire? Probably not unless it's a stormy night and it just so happens to get struck by lightning, which at that point you probably wouldn't want a roasted marshmallow as you yourself will probably be roasted. <u>Proper steps</u> must be taken to ensure a mouth-watering s'more. Right?

Okay, so now that you know the primitive reflexes come from the brain stem, let's talk about this.

First of all, a reflex is an involuntary or unconscious response to a stimulus. In a baby's case, these reflexes start while they are in the womb to help protect the baby and prepare for the birthing process. Sometimes, these little reflex helpers get messed up for several reasons that have been observed over the years:

1. Lots of stress put on the mother during pregnancy, which releases adrenaline and large amounts of adrenaline can cause a baby's system to be very sensitive. Adrenaline in large amounts is also corrosive and can affect the central nervous system in all of us.

2. Eating the foods that the food manufacturers keep putting bad junk into such as hormones, GMO's (genetically modified organisms), MSG, spraying the food with pesticides, etc. thus creating a platform for several of the diseases and syndromes we are seeing today. Why do you think there is such a large rise in autism, allergies, and genetic disorders? I'll get to diet later on.

3. Cell phones, microwaves, computers . . . yes, the waves that come off of them are messing things up. For example, if a man keeps his cell phone in his pocket next

to his scrotum, these waves can affect sperm health as well as sperm count. This is real, I'm not kidding.

4. C-sections! If you don't absolutely have to have a C-section, DO NOT HAVE ONE! This is, in my opinion, one of THE top reasons why these reflexes are being retained. Not every C-section, but the majority of them. The vaginal birthing process gets the crank turning if you will, and out comes the reflexes to aid in the birthing process, thus launching the proper order of things. When a C-section is done, those reflexes get all confused like how you would feel if you accidentally walked into the wrong bathroom at a restaurant and saw a man's hinny that was not your husband's/boyfriend's or men, you walked in on a chick pulling down her shirt in the mirror having just finished adjusting 'the girls,' it throws you, right? Although really, some of you men are kind of freaky and you'd probably take a pause and stare, I'm just saying. Anyway, it'll disorient you a bit and in the case of reflexes, it can mess them up a little or a lot depending on the platform that is being built. I'll touch more on this 'platform' I am referring to in a bit.

5. If you had a severe viral infection while you were pregnant during the first 12 weeks or between 26 and 30 weeks. This can also cause autism, though it's not the only way. I'll get to that later on too.

6. Drinking or drugs while pregnant. Don't drink please and certainly don't do drugs while you're pregnant or anytime for that matter.

7. If you were exposed to radiation.

8. Uncontrolled diabetes-get your check-ups!

9. Smoking . . . okay, really, don't smoke!

10. If you had hypertension or high blood pressure during your pregnancy-go to your check-ups.

11. A traumatic birth, I'll explain in a bit.

12. Undiagnosed thyroid disease, which may be coming from a virus and/or your liver. I'll explain this later.

13. And yes, the vaccinations that we got as babies can affect our children. I may be killed by the drug

companies for saying this but it is the truth! I'll go into detail on this later because it needs to be said.

Now, the only thing on this list that is your fault is drinking, drugs, smoking, you didn't go to your checkups, therefore, neglecting to know that you had high blood pressure or diabetes, or a thyroid issue, but I guess if you couldn't afford to go then I'll digress on that one, although there are some free clinics out there, just saying.

I had a new precious little girl on my caseload a few weeks back and God bless her she has a mess of retained reflexes but we are working on them and she's making lovely progress. So much progress in fact that when she came to me at nearly 36 months old, her physical therapist (PT) told her mom that she was functioning at about a 15-month-old level, physically. After I saw her for one month, she went back for her final evaluation from her PT, because she aged out of early intervention, and lo and behold, she had shot up to a 23-month age equivalency! IN 1 MONTH!!!

When I met my sweet OT kid and her mother for the first time, the mom explained the way this poor child was born and I nearly threw up all over my clinic.

Here's why . . .

Picture this . . . its New Year's Eve and someone has just suggested some lovely bubbly and as you stand there watching, you see that the opening-of-the-bottle individual is struggling to get that dang cork out. He's grunting and straining, oh, and oops, he just farted to boot, bless him, and finally, he yanks the sucker out and it hits the ceiling. The sound of the cork being sucked out of the bottle is a familiar one if you have ever had wine or champagne.

Now, picture this . . . your doctor has just announced that a C-section is going to have to be done because the baby is in trouble, you agree, reluctantly but you do, birthing docs will sometimes treat you as if there are no other choices so you panic and agree. Remember that cork getting yanked out?

As the sweet mom describes it, they did the unsavory cutting of her belly and as they were trying to get this tiny baby out, she was in an awkward position and was a bit stuck . . . you see where I'm going with this. Not only did the C-section mess up the whole reflexes falling into place gig, but the doc also had to literally put his foot on the bed, grab this child by a body part, and pulled that cork-like baby out of her mother with that fun cork-coming-out-suction sound. The force they applied to get this child out, literally violently jostled the whole bed her mother told me. Can you even imagine what this did to that poor baby? What an unbelievable and unnecessary trauma that this child had to endure! Plus, the unfortunate snowball effect it has had on her, her retained reflexes, her development, but especially, especially the guilt her mom had and the counseling she had to go through to get over what had happened.

This woman is now a part of a group that educates the general public about the dangers a C-section can have on a child and that women have a choice!

Now, OBGYN people, I completely understand that I have not walked in your flip-flops for miles and I <u>don't</u> completely understand your emotional level or what is going on in your mind with a screaming woman in front of you or the nature of every situation, I don't claim to and I won't claim to, however, you practitioners know who you are. The ones who just decided to take the lazy way out because you had a barbeque to go to later and just wanted this birth over with. You are also the ones convincing these ladies that a C-section is a lot easier on everyone and a C-section baby is 'just beautiful.' Shame on you, you have created a domino effect now stop it right now!

Primitive Reflexes Part 2

All right, what in the heck are these primitive reflexes the crazy Southern OT lady keeps talking about? Well, hold your horses' people we are here now for that very thing!

Reflexes were designed to protect the baby in its mom's belly, aid in the birthing process, hang out for a bit to help with development such as rolling over, crawling, eating, etc., and then when their turn is over, they mosey on back to the brain stem and shut the heck up. Overall, these primitive reflexes should be integrated at around 7 months but a few of them don't integrate until around 12-18 months.

Well, as you can see, this doesn't always happen. Sometimes these reflexes act like that insane relative, we will call her Aunt Edna, that just won't stop talking to you at the family reunion as you go into a catatonic-like state and wish for anywhere but here. It's time for her to move on!

These reflexes HAVE to go away when it's time because they can wreak havoc on the process of development and we now have an idea of what may cause them to retain. Let's talk about what they are and if retained, what they can look like. Also, at the end of this book, in the Appendix, I have included an at-home checklist for you to fill out and go over with your health care doctor, counselor, and/or your OT, PT, and/or speech therapist (ST).

Now, I can give you all the when-its-suppose-to-be-integrated-hoopla exactly, but that doesn't hugely matter at this point. I've got to give you the meat, not all the garnish. Who the heck eats that garnish anyway?

Moving on . . .

The Fear Paralysis Reflex

This is a reflex that the baby has in the womb. This reflex is a protective one for mom and baby. This is what I tell my OT kids: "Okay, let's say mom is just coming out of the grocery store pregnant with you and she looks up and says, "Oh sweet baby Jesus, that is a tornado and it's coming this way!" Two things happen to her; well several so wait for it. First, 2 chemicals that we know of are released when there is a fearful situation for a mom who is pregnant or even not pregnant, actually; they are adrenalin and cortisol. When these get out into her circulatory system, it goes into the umbilical cord and into the baby's system." So, some of the OT kids will always ask, "Well what grocery store is she at," and when I look at them, I say, "Um, kid you are missing the point, keep listening." So, I then say, "Now, does it make more sense for you to be still or flailing like a crazy baby with your arms and legs kicking and screaming in there in case she has to run?" Every one of them gets this answer right, I just love kids, they are so cool.

This inherently makes sense to every kid I tell this story to. That baby freezes because the mother has to protect both of them and doesn't need little freaked out Johnny kicking and screaming in there distracting her from the immediate task at hand or knocking her off balance as she is running because of the flailing. She is in survival mode for both so the baby remains still to help her get everyone to safety.

<u>If retained, the following may occur:</u>

1. Seems to have high anxiety overall

2. Poor self-esteem

3. Sleep or eating disorders/issues

4. Above necessary aggression

5. Fear of failure or embarrassment

6. Unexplained phobias

7. Extremely jumpy, doesn't like loud sounds, panic attacks

An aside, my now-husband aka the Professor has this one, he'll probably kick my hinny for mentioning it, but I want you to know that this can happen to OTs too and adults and everyone, really.

We think his has come back out because of the trauma of the divorce from his first wife. Plus, the exit of two of his kids out of the house 2 weeks apart from each other and the sorrow that followed. One went off to college and the other went back to live with her mother out of nowhere.

An aside, as a child, teenager, or adult, primitive reflexes can pop back out if there is a traumatic and/or emotional event in one's life. Crazy, I know, but true.

This retained reflex of his has caused a domino effect in his life. He is afraid of heights, he's claustrophobic big time, and he has anxiety attacks. However, he is being treated by me, his personal OT, and is making gains!!! He's 52 years old and making gains! Just another example of the plasticity of the brain all through our lives!

The Moro Reflex

The other name for this one is the Startle Reflex. A <u>newborn</u> baby is incapable of rational thought and therefore, God gave it an alarm reflex, which is triggered by excessive information to any of its senses. A loud noise, a bright light, sudden rough touch, or like I tell the OT kids, "Okay, let's say mom is holding you and your silly sausage older brother has dropped something off of his high chair, so mom leans over to pick it up and your head gently rocks back a bit. Here's what you will do, your little arms will flail out away from your body and so will your little feet so you will look like a starfish for a second but then you will close in like a ball (fetal position) to protect your core aka your heart." Of course, there's always that one kid that asks, "Well, what did the silly sausage big brother drop on the floor that would make my mom bend over to pick it up and rock back my head like that?" Oh, these crazy children . . . I always tell them it was just a piece of sausage and then they launch into,

"Well is it cut small so my brother doesn't choke, what kind, is it mild or spicy". . . oh Lord help this OT! I LOVE MY JOB TO BITS!

If retained, the following may occur:

1. Carsickness, poor balance, and poor coordination

2. Poor stamina

3. Does not maintain eye contact

4. Sensitive to light

5. Sensitive to sound

6. Allergies

7. Adverse reactions to drugs

8. Hypoglycemia

9. Strong dislikes to change

10. Anxiety or nervousness

11. Mood swings

12. Poor math sense

I have this retained reflex, as you read at the beginning of this book when I described high school, and it is not fun at all. I get very carsick and airsick and in a real-life situation here's an example of the domino effect that can happen: I don't fly unless it is ABSOLUTELY necessary and only with my friend Dramamine, I may never see parts of the world that look so interesting to me, I prefer to drive (that's dang tiring and stressful especially this past beach trip, don't get me started), I hate loud sudden sounds, if someone decides it's time to get their kicks and giggles on and scare me (my son), well, it's very very ugly. As I mentioned at the beginning of this book, I thought I was claustrophobic but what was actually happening was the retention of this reflex. What I mean is that, for me, crowds were unpredictable therefore, I would panic a little in response to the unknown of someone scaring the crud out of me or jostling/bumping into me, for example. I am doing my reflex integrating exercises but it takes time, though it's a lot better.

So, you see, these retained reflexes follow you around and affect your quality of life, hold you back from things you want to do but don't feel like you can, and it sucks, it really does.

Incidentally, the Moro Reflex is the earliest form of the adrenal 'fight or flight response' and prepares for fighting or fleeing. This retained reflex can look like hyperactivity as well because of the constant fight or flight challenge in the body or like I tell my OT kids and parents, "You are like always humming inside, like a hummingbird who is always rapidly moving those little wings." Also, the adrenal glands are a large part of our immune system and each time they are stimulated, because of the retained reflex, it can lead to adrenal fatigue and therefore issues such as asthma, allergies, autoimmune diseases, and chronic illness.

Let's think about the rise in autoimmune diseases for a minute. If too much cortisol and adrenalin are floating around in your system all the time because of this retained reflex, you will also gain weight or have a hard time losing it, you can lose all of your hair as I did because of a disease similar to alopecia called telogen effluvium, you are more prone to a heart attack, and I've read recently that's why we women and men have that stinking belly fat, though it can be from a fatty and sluggish liver, I'll get to that.

At this point, you are probably thinking, "Well, heck these first two explain a lot about that freakish relative, Aunt Edna, that insists on talking to me at the reunion and jumps every time someone bangs a dish, and really, she just always seems so generally freaked out and it freaks me out!" Yes people, perhaps she has both of these retained reflexes as well.

Babkin (not Babinski) Reflex

So, remember when you were nursing your baby or giving him/her a bottle and their little hands started clenching and releasing? In other words, as they were sucking, their hands were moving. The other thing you may have noticed is that a baby's mouth opens before its hand reaches it during play. Hence, the baby or toddler putting everything in their mouth, it's also one of the most nerve-ending ridden parts of the body (next to our crotches), and gives babies a lot of input and information about an object. This can drive parents insane, especially if it is a snake or large roach, just kidding, but it could happen. Mom says I tried to eat a roach that had crawled out of the newspaper and onto my high chair as a baby . . . good times!

If retained, the following may occur:

1. Tendency to clutch fists when unnecessary with thumb tucked into the palm (I see a lot in the clinic)

2. Hyper-mobility in the fingers

3. Sensitivities in the palms of the hands

4. Difficulties with overall fine-motor skills/handwriting/fasteners/eating utensils

5. Moves tongue, lips, or mouth involuntarily when using hands such as in handwriting

6. Speech and articulation issues

7. Under-developed facial expressions

8. Tension in the jaw and tooth grinding

9. Regularly chews pencils, fingernails, etc.

I had this one too and chewed the stew out of pen tops, gum (especially in college), I ALWAYS had my tongue out when writing or doing anything else that took effort, and I was always balling my fists to where my hands would ache.

At this point you are probably thinking, wait a dang minute, I think I have this retained reflex stuff too? Yep, you just might but you've made it this far and you have a family and a couple of kids so you've done good, and remember, human beings have tenacity and plasticity of the brain.

The other thing to think about . . . struggle builds character and we human beings are very adaptable and have lots of ingenuity and grit. I mean, my ADHD was a 10 on the scale, but I managed to graduate from college with a 4.0 and un-medicated to boot!

The Rooting Reflex

This reflex is seen when your tiny baby gets stimulation on the corner of its mouth and then turns toward the stimulated side, opens its mouth, and extends its tongue to prepare for suckling. It helps the baby get the nipple in its mouth whether it's boob or bottle.

An aside . . . for my first few years as a pediatric OT, I saw older kids like 9 and 10 still drooling while they were at the clinic doing their work. This baffled me and I couldn't figure out why drool kept coming out of these big kid's mouths and they didn't seem to notice it at all. What was happening was if something brushed their cheek/corner of their mouth while doing their session, it would trigger salivation. I'll get to all the things I do for this stuff a bit later, although you really do need an OT to do a full evaluation because there might be other things going on, not just retained reflexes. I'll get to that too.

If retained, the following may occur:

1. Picky eater

2. Continues to suck thumb at an older age

3. Often drool dribbles from his/her mouth

4. Speech and articulation issues

So, keep this reflex in mind if you have a picky eater and there are a lot of them out there. Speech Therapists and Occupational Therapists see this ALL the time and I know it freaks you parents out when your kid is so picky you fear they will starve to death. The other thing that happens is they are usually carb crazies, right? I'll give you an explanation of why these kids are carb crazies later on.

So, you give them those hormone riddled fake chicken nuggets because you are so dang tired of listening to them refuse everything you cook but hark, now you've just added gas to fire because hormones, GMO's, and pesticides may have been injected in these foods, and wreaks havoc on the body, the gut, and these reflexes. We will talk about diet later on.

Palmar Reflex

If you have ever been around a newborn baby, you have probably noticed that when you put your finger in the palm of their hand, they wrap their tiny fingers around it as if they are holding your finger. This is the Palmar or Grasp Reflex and I'm terribly sorry to burst your little bubble when you say, "Oh my Lord, the tiny baby is holding onto my finger! Can you believe that? What a smart kid!" It's a reflex folks, sorry.

Anyway, this reflex is essential for developing fine-motor skills, sensory input, and this fancy Nancy word called stereognosis, which in layman's terms means, the ability you use to reach into your purse groping for your keys without looking at your hand or in your purse, you can just feel that you have them in your hand once you have found them.

Not sure if any of you younger parents remember this but this reflex reminds me of a show that was on 100 years ago called 'Mutual of Omaha' with that old dude with white hair and that little salt and pepper mustache who had these cool African shows about the animals that roamed the plains there.

Remember how those little baby chimps would grasp onto their mom's fur if she bent over or had to walk off somewhere? I think this is where this reflex stems from when we were evolving and still had body hair. Our babies used this reflex to hold the heck on when we were on the move and yes, I believe in the big bang theory and the story of evolution, but of course, God caused all of it.

An aside, scientists have now admitted that our universe, stars, planets, Earth, people, nature, etc. has too much complexity to be 'started' by any 'sciencey' thing or person as it is bigger than science. Of course, it's God, wake the heck up. If you've ever grown a whole child in your belly and watched them pop out, vaginally hopefully, you know there is a God. Just watch that movie 'The Shack' if you don't believe me, it will teach you a thing or two . . . oh, and get your tissues, you'll need them.

If retained, the following may occur:

1. Poor handwriting

2. Poor fine-motor skills overall

3. A less than functional pencil grip, therefore fatiguing the hand quicker

4. Poor posture when using the hands

5. Difficulty putting ideas in their heads down onto paper

Plantar Reflex

The Plantar Reflex occurs with the stroking or pressing on the bottom of the foot, which causes the foot to flex and the toes to curl, like going back to your monkey days to grasp a banana with your foot. This reflex relates to the movement and coordination of the small foot muscles that will help with many of the gross movements yet to come.

Once your baby starts to stand and then walks, its uber important for this reflex to go away because, in walking, you need your foot to move in the opposite direction of picking up that banana, you need for it to move away from that flexed pattern so you can push off with the bottom of your foot and not kick this reflex into gear. Otherwise, you will have trouble walking and run like some flailing crazy person, well, not really but you'll run awkwardly and uncomfortably and be prone to falls.

An aside, the whole objective of our developing bodies, now think about this and picture it in your mind, is to move <u>away</u> from our core or our trunk as we all start out flexed in a fetal position. Think of it like a rosebud.

Now, if you stay a bud and never bloom away from your closed-up self, you will not be able to utilize your full potential as a beautiful rose bloom. A flower that stays a bud has missed its full potential. The job of our bodies is to move away from our core and bloom out and away from it and be the beautiful 'rose' we are all capable of being.

Now, can a bud grow and bloom without water? Can a bud grow and bloom without the sun? No, you, mom and dad or mom and mom or dad and dad, are the water and the sun and I am the pruner to give your 'bud' the best-blooming potential out there and no, OT's do not cut things off of your children, well at least not this

OT, bleh! You get the picture I'm sure, if not, contact me, please.

Moving on . . .

If retained, the following may occur:

1. Difficulty with learning to walk

2. Runs awkwardly

3. Poor balance

4. Since the toes may curl under if the foot is stimulated, putting shoes on may drive you to unrest with your child because this retained reflex will make this hard

5. Problems playing sports that's why I said, "Don't force the sports because they may have this retained reflex and until that is integrated you and they will be frustrated!"

6. Shin soreness

7. Recurrent sprained ankles

8. Difficult walking in the dark where their vision is not there to help with balance.

Asymmetrical Tonic Neck Reflex

All right, this little reflex aka ATNR is the start of a baby's ability to roll over. So here's what you'll see while they are lying in their crib on their back: their head will turn to one side and then their little arms go up like a check-mark, the arm will straighten out on the side their head is turned, and the other arm will bend up with their little hand by their head . . . eventually, this position urges the rolling over of the little baby's body.

One of my OT kids calls it 'dabbing' but without the head tuck to the bent arm side. If you are unfamiliar with dabbing, Google it, it's a crazy move these silly kids do and every time one of them does it in the clinic I say, "Quit making an excuse to smell your armpit already." They laugh every time.

So basically, this is the rolling over helper reflex. Also, note, this reflex is one where the arms and hands move in conjunction with the head so as a result if retained, it can cause a kid to have a lot of trouble looking up to the board in class and copying something down on their paper because of that connection. Remember, a reflex is an involuntary response to a stimulus meaning, you can't stop it once it kicks in.

If retained, the following may occur:

1. Eye-hand coordination issues

2. Poor handwriting

3. Awkward pencil grip

4. Trouble copying from the board

5. Skipping lines or words when reading

6. Trouble catching a ball

7. Not crossing body midline consistently

8. Messes up visual tracking, which in turn, messes up reading

9. Right/left discrimination trouble

10. Trouble establishing a dominant hand, eye, or foot

An aside, my mother has this retained reflex so driving with her is not at all entertaining because when she turns her head to look at something, her whole car via the steering wheel, decides to go in the direction that her head is turned. She's nearly run off the road a number of times. I love her, but she's got to do the exercises I've given her or someone is going to end up in a ditch!

Tonic Labyrinthine Reflex

There are two parts to this reflex aka the TLR that involves the vestibular system, which is that tiny 3-

ring circus inside our ears that was designed to let our brain know where our head is in space. I tell the OT kids it's their 'dizzy' system. They get that.

Anyway, this reflex has to do with the head going forward, like looking at your toes or going backward, like looking up in the sky for Jesus. Now, when your baby does this, you will see something happening to their legs and arms. Looking up, you will see their legs and arms flex out and away from their core. Likewise, when they look down, the arms and legs flex into their core like the fetal position.

Just a quick and further explanation . . . if there is a retained 'forward,' you will see a kid who is very 'floppy.' On the other hand, if you see a retained 'backward' of this reflex, you will see a very rigid and awkward kid with stiff and jerky type movements. I see this retained reflex a lot and if you have a kid who is having trouble going up or down steps, this is probably why. Think about it, as they are coming down the steps, they look down, right, especially if they are new at steps?

What do the legs want to do? Flex, right? Um, is that a good feeling when you need leg extension in unison with flexion to manage the stairs? Probably not.

If retained, the following may occur:

1. A floppy child

2. Poor balance

3. Motion sickness

4. Orientation and spatial difficulties

5. Visual issues

6. Difficulty judging space, distance, depth, and speed

7. Poor concentration

8. Fatigue while reading or working or studying at a desk

9. Bad posture when sitting at a desk

10. Difficulty coordinating movements

11. Not so good at sports

Again, if your kid is not the sport type you dreamed of them being and you are trying to live vicariously through them and they have retained reflexes that are not addressed, you are like a dog chasing its tail, it's not going to happen. Lay off that kid and take them to see a therapist who knows how to help retained reflexes, then let's see what can happen or find something else they can embrace and love!

An aside, so many folks want to focus on the inability of their child, stop that right now! Try focusing on their abilities and you begin to build a confident child.

Spinal Galant

I would call this one the root of a misdiagnosing of ADHD for a lot of kids who get stuck with this 'label.' No one bothered to look at all of the primitive reflexes that are lurking about having not been integrated.

This particular reflex is believed to be very active during the birthing process because of its side-to-side nature when stimulated.

Here's what I mean, if you run a fingertip down just left of the spinal column from the bottom tip of the shoulder blade to the small of the back, you will see a moving of the lower back away from the stimulated side or left side in this case and the left hip will lift as well. Reverse all of that for the right-side fingertip-down scenario. In other words, they will wiggle side to side.

In some children, stimulation down each side at the same time can cause them to pee, not kidding. Please don't tell your kids this or slumber parties for that unfortunate stomach sleeper who may have this retained reflex and fell asleep first, could get a bit damp. This is why it is believed that bedwetting occurs because the sheets simultaneously stimulate each side, which causes urination. Isn't this stuff so interesting?!!!

<u>If retained, the following may occur:</u>

1. The child who **CANNOT** sit still and fidgets and wiggles in their chair as if they have ants in their pants because the back of their chair is stimulating this reflex. I often tell their teachers to get them a stool with no back to help with this.

2. Attention and concentration problems

3. Difficulty coordinating a normal walking gait

4. Bladder control/bedwetting

5. Can be a contributor to scoliosis

6. May affect the efficiency of movement with physical activities or sports.

An aside, my son and daughter both have this one, though they were both born vaginally, but luckily on the retained reflex scale that I use of 0 to 4 in severity, they were both about a 2. It took my daughter a bit to stop wetting the bed at night and she had to wear pull-up for a lot longer than I would have liked but we got it figured out for her and now she is square at 18 years old. Good Lord, finally . . . just kidding, it didn't take that long.

Symmetrical Tonic Neck Reflex

So, let's say you have this baby, ok, and they are on the floor on their belly, you may notice that when they move their chin down towards their chest, their knees will bend up a bit and if they move their head up and back, their legs will straighten. This reflex is the start of learning to crawl on all fours or in 'quadruped.'

Now, again, not to burst bubbles, YOUR KIDS NEED TO CRAWL ON ALL FOURS WITH HEAD UP AND NOT THE COMANDO CRAWL! If your child did not crawl, that does not mean he's some gross-motor advanced genius, that means his reflexes are messed up some, and at some point when you get that inkling that things aren't just right, go out and find yourself a good therapist who knows a lot about retained reflexes so you can cut to the chase of development.

If retained, the following may occur:

1. A child crawling later than normal or not at all

2. Poor hand-eye coordination

3. An ape-like walking pattern

4. Tendency to slump at their desk or in a chair because of under-developed back muscles from not crawling

5. Poor organization and planning skills

Stepping Reflex and Heel Reflex

Our bodies alter our posture depending on if the weight is over our heels or our toes. The Stepping and Heel Reflexes are believed to help remove tension from the muscles of the lower leg to allow for increased ankle movement. It also helps with ideal posture integrated with vision. These two reflexes serve to balance the connection between the input from our eyes and the feedback from our feet.

If the Stepping Reflex is retained, the following may occur:

1. Toe walking

2. Tight calves

3. Poor balance and muscle control

4. Feet and ankle problems with pain and dysfunction

5. Recurring hamstring injuries and mid-low back strains

6. Visual problems due to an altered perception of the horizon-head tilts forward and eyes look up

If the Heel Reflex is retained, the following may occur:

1. Heavy heel walking

2. Heel pain

3. Achilles tendonitis

4. Shin splints

5. Poor core stability

6. Balance problems

7. Visual problems due to an altered perception of the horizon-head tilts back and eyes look down

An aside, I had this heel one as a child and it integrated itself. I couldn't sneak up on a deaf person without them turning around because of the tremendous vibration of my very heavy heel walking. Funny thing, my daughter is a heavy heel walker too and to pin her down to do her exercises is like pinning down the wind. Oh well, maybe hers will integrate as mine did.

Sometimes they just do that but it depends on the level/severity.

Suprapubic Reflex

So, you may go into the mental gutter, where I went, when I learned of this particular reflex but funny thing is, one of my OT kids has this and I just thought he was humping the floor and self-stimulating his boy parts. Self-stimulation is seen a lot in what I do and not all self-stimulation is bad, society can be very judgy and make us think we have to correct every cotton pickin' thing about our kids. Let me tell you something, we all self-stimulate or self-regulate in some way. For example, if I have to sit through a lecture, as sitting still for me is torture, you better believe that my leg is either bouncing or if my leg is crossed, kicking up a storm. If your kid is a flapper of the hands, leave them alone because they need to do this and to take that away is like taking oxygen away from them.

So, this reflex is very interesting and I remember this one as a teenager and I know that may sound like TMI or too much information thing for you but when I share, I open myself up to others to accept or not accept, and maybe they have this too and now feel that they are not alone.

This reflex is elicited when pressure is detected at the pubic bones and the body responds by tipping the pelvis forward and both legs straighten out. Now, think about this and 'dry humping,' I know, but I'm giving you easy-to-understand stuff here, so bear with me, okay?

So, you are getting happy with your husband, boyfriend, or significant other fully clothed (I will keep it clean). You are on the bottom and there's a bit of 'junk' rubbing together, what do our hips do when that junk rubs above or very near our pubic bone area? Yep, we tilt our pelvis up and yes, our legs may straighten.

Now, there may be research out there that I have not come across that would call this some sexual response to a stimulus and not this Suprapubic reflex, and okay, yes, maybe. I just wanted to throw it out there, as I have seen this kid hump the floor right before he has to pee or poo, believe it or not. Read on for this last bit to make sense. Anyway, if anyone has something to add to this one, I'd be open to listening. There is a bit more to this reflex actually so I'll throw it out there.

If the actual skin of the baby is touched above the pubic bone you will see one hip moving forward and the other one moves back as well as the opposite pattern in the upper body and when all put together, this initiates the commando crawling before the Symmetrical Tonic Neck Reflex activates but eh, okay. I don't want to get terribly deep here.

I looked some stuff up and found this . . . this reflex is greatly correlated with kidney function/health, pelvic floor tone, and bladder control/health. Scientists also have linked it to the most ancient part of our brains called the hypothalamus, which controls body temperature, appetite, sexual pleasure, hence the dry humping I mentioned, and the glandular activity in the body, which regulates our very unique biochemistry.

Again, this one is a weirdo but I felt it was worth mentioning especially if you have a floor-humping child, this may be why. He/she may be using this reflex to get him/herself to pee or poo. I have a lot of kids that hold their poo, maybe I should teach this private in-your-home way to initiate it perhaps. Stay tuned on that one.

<u>If retained, the following may occur</u>:

1. Bladder problems

2. Pelvic floor problems

3. Sugar handling imbalances

4. Imbalances in the hormone system

5. May affect walking pattern and posture

6. Difficult or reoccurring ankle, hip, and shoulder problems

The website that I have learned a lot from is out of Australia and those folks have it going on and I pray to the good Lord above I will have enough money to fly over there someday, heavily medicated so I don't know I'm flying I guess and learn from them but alas, I'm not rolling in it. I often see kids who don't have insurance at a very very low out-of-pocket charge or sometimes even for free because I can't turn kids or families away.

I remember years ago learning that if you didn't help a person in need, you could be turning away Jesus Himself and that has stuck with me all of my life. My payment will hopefully be in heaven someday, that is if I'm worthy.

****

The reflexes that I have just explained are the ones that I felt were worth mentioning because these affect the developing child and their little worlds physically, academically, spiritually, emotionally, and socially all the way through pre-school, elementary school, middle school, high school, college, and then eventually out there in the real world.

Sometimes these retained reflexes are misdiagnosed and labeled **ADHD**, oppositional defiance, Asperger's, and many more in my professional opinion. Sometimes these kids, including me at one time, are called 'quirky' or low IQ or trouble or problematic or mean or whatever the heck else they decide to label us. I hate labels because they can limit the definition we have for ourselves and force us into a box, not of our own making. Here is what I say to that, get the box cutter and bust out kids because you are way more than what you are being told, heck we all are!

Another thing I want to mention is that I have a lot of parents that come to me about their child needing OT services and ask me if I want to see all of the paperwork that has ever been cranked out on their kid from past therapies to counseling or even medical exams like MRI's, spinal taps, etc. and I always politely say this,

"No, I don't care about all that hooey, I want to use the freedom of my own eyes, my own mind, my own heart, and my own intuitive neurons that God gave me to get a feel for your child. Don't give me all the labels that they have 'bestowed' on your child either, I am fresh eyes, I do not judge, I am the person that will help them soar using my Dragonfly Approach. However, this is not to say that I don't take heed to any precautions or allergies."

There have been tears after I have said this and a sparkle of renewed hope in the eyes of these parents. This junk that many of the doctors, some of the therapists, some of the counselors, and definitely the internet and media tell them, freaks them out or ignores their cries for any kind of help to understand what is going on with their child, and it has GOT TO STOP!

It is time to be empowered, parents and kids. Let me help you get to the bottom of what is really going on and to also better understand yourselves as human beings on this awesome planet we have been given. The time is now!

Oh, and once again, I am sick and dang tired of docs throwing meds at all of these kids and not getting to the root of the problem. Shame on you, that's lazy doctoring if you ask me. There is a new breed of doctors out there called Functional Medicine Doctors who are looking at the whole person emotionally, medically, physically, and spiritually. It's about time.

I also recommend looking into hooking your family up with a board-certified Naturopathic Doctor who approaches things naturally and is also eager to get to the root of the problem if you can't find a Functional Medical Doctor in your area. I also feel the need to say that not all doctors outside of the aforementioned are bad or don't listen, there is just a certain number that seems to just want to make their paycheck and go home. That's just not fair to these kids. Don't work with kids just to make a paycheck!

Reflex Integrating Exercises

In this chapter, I was going to take some snappy pictures of my daughter in the various positions for each exercise but because it is a book, I think videos are way better. I thought about making my own but there are some great videos on YouTube and some of the channels that I like and refer my OT kids to are as follows:

1. The Adah Company

2. Pyramid of Potential

3. The Organized Mind

4. Pediatric Potentials

5. Whatif244

6. Michelle Kyle

7. Psalmseeker

8. Raina Koterba

9. Elizabeth Jones-Twomey

Another interesting therapy that helps integrate these retained reflexes is called Rhythmic Movement Therapy. This therapy is based on the work of a gal named Kerstin Linde who is a Swedish movement specialist. She developed these movements based on how babies move. This therapy is a series of gentle rocking and reflex integration movements that stimulate nerve pathways and promote emotional balance, learning, and ease of movement. It is a very effective way to help with not only integrating reflexes but also helps with symptoms of ADHD/ADD, learning disabilities, autism, and emotional issues without the use of drugs. For more information and resources on this type of therapy please refer to this website: rhythmicmovement.org.

****

I have recently run across a treatment for retained reflexes in the form of cold laser therapy, specifically red-light therapy, which penetrates the deepest.

The reason the laser is called 'cold' is that it penetrates the skin with no heating effect or tissue damage and the awesome thing is that the laser can penetrate the skin up to 2+ inches, which produces a photochemical effect that promotes healing and cellular organization.

Photons, the basic unit of light emitted by the cold laser, stimulate cellular mitochondria to increase the production of adenosine triphosphate or ATP. Faster healing time is the result because ATP is considered the 'battery' or the energy source for the cell.

ATP governs about 85% of cellular activity, including 'replication.' Replication is "the process by which a double-stranded DNA molecule is copied to produce two identical DNA molecules." Replication is necessary for replacing cells that have died and in keeping our cellular supply at the necessary level for our overall health. Thus, cold laser therapy can be used for several other areas as well such as anti-aging, muscle gain, pain, performance, and recovery.

If you have ever heard of or experienced acupuncture, you probably know about 'acupoints' or energy points along the meridians of the body. This cold laser unit can be used instead of needles, which may be very beneficial to those kids and adults that get freaked out by needles and works a lot quicker.

In other words, a cold laser unit works by stimulating the cells and improving natural healing which can take the place of steroids and other synthetic medications. With regards to, retained reflexes, cold laser therapy guides and helps integrate them back into the brain stem.

Meridians are associated with acupoints…it is best to consider the meridians of the body as an energetic distribution network within itself that tends towards energetic manifestation. Meridians can be best understood as a process rather than a structure.

Basic substances of the body like Qi (Chee), blood, and body fluids permeate the whole body by way of these meridians. Qi can be defined as the circulating life force whose existence and properties are the basis of much Chinese philosophy and medicine.

Okay, now that I've completely gone south with all of this, I challenge you to think outside of Western Medicine and look this stuff up. It's real and the folks of Western Medicine tried to shove this natural way of being a human aside making it look like God had designed our bodies in a flawed manner. Modern man aka doctors, make us believe that they were put on this earth to throw meds at an ill-designed body of God's doing. I know I'm getting deep but look this up. Better yet, I challenge you to look up the book 'The Drug Story' by Morrison Allison Bealle and then tell me I'm full of you know what.

Ancient healing is not hooey, but the beginning of Western Medicine decided that drugs made money so all of the natural ways of healing our bodies needed to be squashed such as the areas of acupuncture, meditation, Reiki healing, essential oils, etc. I'll step down here but you would be sick to know what the underlying push was to get meds into our bodies whether they worked or not.

There is a new movement that is slowly coming about, which describes the necessity of marrying Western and Eastern health ideas as they can actually complement each other because I will admit, there are a lot of life-saving advancements that Western Medicine does offer. Now, fancy that, folks cooperating with each other for the greater good of man and not for the greed of man!

Sensory Integration aka Sensory Processing Disorder

Sensory integration is our body's ability to process all of the input that comes in through all 7 to 21 or senses as neurologists are uncovering several more here lately. First off, the definition of 'sense' is any system that consists of a group of sensory cell types that respond to a very specific physical event and that corresponds to a specific group of areas within the brain where the signals are received and interpreted. Most folks think of the basic 5 senses but there appears to be a lot more.

Here are a few:

*Hearing or auditory

*Touch or tactile

*Visual or visual

*Taste or gustatory

*Smell or olfactory

*Pressure

*Itch

*Thermoception- the ability to sense hot and cold

*Tension Sensors-the sensors for muscle tension

*Equilibrioception-the sense that allows you to keep your balance with directional and accelerative change

*Stretch Receptors-these are found in such areas as lungs, bladder, stomach, and gastrointestinal tract

*Chemoreceptors-simplified, this one is involved in the vomiting reflex

*Hunger

*Time-this one is debated at the moment but some folks have a heightened awareness of time and scientists are curious about this

And the ones that I tap into a lot in my practice are:

*Vestibular-this is the system located in the inner ear, it's that 3 ring circus I told you about that lets the brain knows where the head is in space. Again, I tell the kids it's their 'dizzy' system.

*Proprioception-this is the system/receptors located in the joints and muscle bellies that lets the brain know where the body is in space. It's the system that lets your hand that sippy cup back to your child in the back seat of the car without having to watch your hand take the journey to the back seat; you just know where your arm is without looking. It is also the system that lets you know how hard or soft to hold an egg and also remember the unsavory story I told you of my daughter whose sense of proprioception was off, hence the **RIP** frog?

Our systems can either be under-responsive; like that kid at school that your daughter complains about who is always crashing into the wall or other kids or is even falling out of his seat. He needs a lot of extra input.

Or that other kid who can spin and spin and never seems to gets dizzy, this kid has an under-responsive vestibular system.

Then there's the other side, over-responsive. The kid that does not like to be touched, doesn't like loud sounds, or doesn't like movement and God help her if you try to spin or swing her on a swing.

In the appendix, I have included a thorough sensory integration checklist so you can get a feel for where your child might be with this whole sensory thing. Once you have filled it out, it will give you a better idea of what you are seeing in your child, yourself, or maybe your great Aunt Edna at that reunion who makes you crazy, God bless her.

Some basic signs that your child might be dealing with sensory processing issues include:

-Over or under sensitivity to touch, movement, sights, or sounds

-Specific learning difficulties/delays in academic achievement

-Difficulty making transitions from one situation to another

-The tendency to be easily distracted or have a limited attention span for their age

-Activity level that is unusually high or low

-Social and/or emotional problems

-Difficulty learning new movements

-Delays in speech, language, or oral motor skills

-Physical clumsiness or apparent carelessness

-Impulsive behavior or lacking self-control

-Inability to unwind or calm self

-Poor self-concept/body awareness

-Signs of OCD or obsessive-compulsive disorder, which is often misdiagnosed because if a child's system cannot properly digest, analyze, and spit out the right output, then, of course, a kid is going to line their world up in nice neat 'rows.' They <u>have</u> to because they cannot bear to be surprised by anything that might throw their precious unable-to-process-properly world out of whack thus freaking their system out. They are also hugely resistant to change for this reason.

So, why do you think the children or even ourselves have sensory processing issues and why do you think they are getting worse? Any takers?

Well, think about a couple of things that have vastly changed over the last several years: cell phones, computers, gaming, fast food, a faster overall pace of living, increase in stress, an increase in the junk they are putting in our food, less exercise, convenience, inactivity, an enormous increase in the number of vaccinations that are now being given to children and adults . . . I could go on and on.

My point is we as a society are creating the havoc we so despise or are very worried about in our children. Now, I will not admit to putting any junk aka poison in the food, that's on the food people or the additives that have been put in the vaccinations, shame on you. I will admit to an increase in stress and my reliance on technology, shame on me.

As we have seen, there is a layering of things that keep kids from developing to their full potential and if we don't catch it early, it just makes it that much harder for them. It can also cause that domino effect later in life I spoke of earlier and it can all start even before the parents meet or even get married.

For example, you do some weed because you live in one of those states that have legalized it or you steal it from your naughty illegal using cousin. If you are a man, your sperm count can go down or you can have deformed sperm. If you are a chick doing weed, you can harm your eggs. You were also immunized as a baby.

You get a cell phone, guys stuff it in their pockets near their scrotum, thus affecting their sperm again where women, my friend, in particular, carries her phone in her cross-body purse, which so happens to lie against her body in proximity or on top of her ovaries, and yes, affects her eggs.

Fast-forward some, you've met the man or woman of your dreams, you've started a 'situation' if you will, within your body because of the unsavory choices you previously made. You decide to have kids but along the way, you've been eating the food that the stupid food people have added terrible things to, which adds another layer to the altered chemical make-up of your body.

Lo and behold you become pregnant, and man is your job stressful here lately thus you release large quantities of cortisol and in some cases, adrenalin in your system each day. You eat out a lot because of work, as you just don't have time to pack your lunch. You love eating out but you aren't really sure what GMO'S are and who has ever heard of the negative effects of gluten until recently, really. You also love drinking cow's milk with your new chocolate chip cookie craving you've acquired since being pregnant and on and on. Please say no to cow's milk, as I will explain in the 'Diet' chapter.

The day comes for the birth of your child and your doctor talks you into a planned C-section because the baby will be so much prettier and that way you can plan for things. You agree because you haven't read this book yet. You then have your child immunized.

A platform for chaos has inadvertently been laid and it is my job to destroy this platform once and for all for the future couples of the world or at least lessen it for your next baby or future parents out there having or are planning for their first.

I can't stress enough the importance of avoiding a C-section if at all possible because those reflexes don't get to do the job they were supposed to do for your baby and I tell my parents all of the time that a basic protocol for C-section born babies needs to be an automatic OT and/or PT intervention/evaluation between the ages of

2 months to 2 years old to rule out the possibility of retained reflexes.

These reflexes not getting to do their job would be like having multiple interviews and finally getting that dream job you've always wanted, you go in the first day of work ready to kick butt, and they say, "Um, no, you are mistaken, go home, you don't have a job." What would you feel or think?

Here's what I think, you would walk away defeated and confused and you might even doubt yourself and your ability. Later, you may get really upset and throw a bit of a tantrum about it after finding out that in addition to not having your dream job, you have come down with a cold to boot.

Now, imagine those reflexes and how they feel. They have a job that has been as basic as one-ply toilet paper. They are poised and ready but there's this weird stuff floating around in this system of the pregnant lady and suddenly, the baby goes out the wrong part of the body and they don't get to use the Spinal Galant to wiggle out or some of the other ones that are ready to go.

Yes, these reflexes that don't get to do their job throw a fit of their own and remain present even when the party is over for them and it is time for them to go home. They can't help it! They are ticked! Plus, a platform of irregularity within your body has been built by the various technologies and the waves that come off of them, your pot use, and that blasted junk they are putting in our food, your vaccinations, and also the junk we are breathing in our air. It is a wonder we haven't made ourselves extinct. Although if you have read anything about the ancient Atlanteans, who yes, existed, Google it, we are headed in their same direction! Plus, there is a growing number of women who cannot get pregnant no matter how hard they try. In the next, 15 years, you will see an even bigger rise in this tragedy.

We haven't done that yet but we have managed to create autism, sensory processing disorder, genetic disorders, autoimmune disorders, allergies (especially all of these nut allergies), and many more because of the 'progress' we claim has been made on this Earth. Ha, progress, what a bunch of baloney. If you think about it, there is irony in progress. Progress will always cause a regression somewhere else. Think about this for a time and you will see that this is disturbingly true.

Technological progress and some medical advancements, have been made, sure, but definitely not so much or as much in the developmental understanding of human children's progress and the effects of all of the things I have thus mentioned.

And I must say it again, <u>sensory processing problems are a direct result of retained reflexes and/or your diet and if your therapist does not start with integrating these reflexes first, everyone will get frustrated. The proper order of treatment is key.</u>

I do both at the same time, actually. I teach the reflex integrating exercises to my parents and OT kids that we may have uncovered and have the kids do them several times per week. I usually start my session doing those very reflex integrating exercises to assess what is happening and if they are working, we then swing and spin because this wakes up the brain and opens it up for learning, and I then set up an obstacle course designed for sensory integration if this is an area they need, which they usually do, honestly. I always tell the OT kids that Movement=Learning, that's why we do so much of it in OT. I also wish that certain schools across our nation would recognize the utmost importance of Movement=Learning as they make the absolutely ridiculous decision to take away recess. Shame on you!

Remember when I told you that it is important to work from the brain stem up, well, it is very important.

To sum up, because I get a bit crazy trying to get you every morsel of information I can for you so you can be empowered when you go into that doctor's office that keeps telling you nothing is wrong:

1. A trained therapist must test your child for retained reflexes, however, it is okay to use my checklist in the back of this book and I encourage you to fill it out and

carry it to your doctor, counselor, PT, OT, ST, etc. If they don't know about this stuff, you need to find one that does for this is the root of many of the issues you are seeing in your child.

2. DO NOT blame yourself if you were misinformed about a C-section, okay, just don't go there with yourself. If you did pot, well, I'm telling your mother and don't do it again. If you don't eat well, again the junk in the food isn't your fault, just stop eating badly. Eat clean, your gut and chemical make-up will thank you, and certainly don't feed that junk to your kids. If you get pregnant again you now have some resources to get a little better at it. Trust me, I messed up too. I was pregnant almost 20 years ago. A lot has changed since then.

3. I have not really said this yet, but we are human, we have done weed/drugs (well not me, I was too afraid), we like eating out, we have become part of this booming technological world, we had some wild oats to sew, etc. so don't blame yourself because I guarantee at 18 you weren't thinking ahead to your middle to late '20s or

early '30s about starting a family, no, you were just living the moment and that's okay because our brains don't really work like that so lay off of yourselves.

4. Clean up your diet!!! Again, I will get to this a bit later.

I'm just sharing this information so you know what to do now, what direction to go, and what wisdom to pass down to the generations. Why do you think Occupational Therapists and all the other therapies are here? We are here to save the day and educate and if your therapist is not doing this, find one that will.

In the Appendix at the end of the book, I have included a sensory integration activity list BUT please consult with a therapist before you go diving into some of these areas. Some of them might be contraindicated for your child or require a measured dose and not over-done, meaning, not a good idea depending on your kid's system.

Brain-Body Mapping/Connection or in Our Case, Remapping

Has anyone ever heard of these phrases? I hadn't either until one day, I was fartin' around on the internet making sure my knowledge was up to date when I came across one of the most fascinating books I have ever read. This book is written by Sandra and Matthew Blakeslee and is called 'The Body Has A Mind of Its Own.' Talk about awesome sauce information!

This book has actually helped transform and enhance the way I treat my OT kids in the clinic and it's working! I'm seeing some of the neatest stuff come out of my kids and they are meeting their personal and family goals left and right as well as doing things that are just . . . WOW!

An aside, my whole philosophy in my practice is not meeting goals as if I'm meeting some personal quota of, "Ha, another goal met, I'm so awesome." No, not at all! When I meet a family and the awesome OT kid I have the privilege of working with, there is a huge pow-wow that takes place; this is a major part of my Dragonfly Approach.

First of all, I treat the whole child, not their hand or their eyes or their sensory system . . . the WHOLE child. This is where many therapists get it wrong. Now, I'm not saying I'm perfect and I know all, that's just stupid as heck to even think or better yet, say out loud because arrogance is ugly as sin. What I'm saying is we are not a hand walking around the mall, right? We are not a set of eyes hanging out at the library with our two sets of eyes children, right? We are not a leg watching our leg children play a soccer game, right? Then why in the heck would I not include the entire being as a whole?

Treating the whole child includes treating the family and no, I'm not a family psychologist though I do have a minor in psychology. The thing you have to realize is that each 'being' in a family intermingles all of their feelings, short-comings both mentally, physically, emotionally, and spiritually. Then you add in the special needs kid's stuff like therapy and doctor visits. This family also includes the sibling(s), who doesn't have special needs and often feels shafted because of the lack of attention. This is just the way it is when you have a special needs kid. Then there is all the other junk out there in the world that wiggles its way into their lives bad or good. That's a lot for one little family to handle. This family is literally hardwired into each other's brain maps.

It is my job and duty to not only include my OT kid in my whole child approach . . . . you CANNOT forget the family because believe it or not, they each have stuff they are dealing with too.

So if you were to come into my 'Oz,' as my clinic has been called quite a lot, on your first visit for your initial evaluation, I do a few standardized/measurable tests with your sweet precious child (you see the insurance companies need measurements, they don't look at us as humans or whole humans as they should, we are a number and according to many of them, a burden to their company, I'll step down, sorry, it just ticks me off) and A LOT of observation as that is my very best way to see what's what. I may also throw a sibling in there to play with my new OT kid, because wow, you can see even more. I also watch and listen to the parent(s). Sometimes I don't get an entire evaluation done in one go and that's okay because think about it, this kid has just arrived in Oz and they are a bit distracted and that's okay, heck, so are the parents. I love it.

Once I have gotten as much as I need to complete my evaluation, we have a come to Jesus with the new OT kid, the parents, and the sibling(s). Now you are probably thinking, "Um, aren't these sessions for the OT kid with special needs or issues?" Yes, they are, but, again, what 'group' does this OT kid belong to that is one of the most important groups they will ever be a part of in their entire life?

F-A-M-I-L-Y!

Our pow-wow is this and the order can change depending on the situation:

1. What are your goals mom/dad for your child to have the best quality of life possible? What has their teacher mentioned to you about classroom stuff?

2. Hey, OT kid, what do you want to get better at? You, not your mom, dad, teacher, or your best friend, you. What irritates and makes you the saddest that you can't do well or just want to get better at? Or do you want to learn something new?

3. Sibling(s), what do you want to see your OT kid sibling be able to do with you like ride bikes with you or play house with you? (This is where you will see a sibling start feeling really important and not so left out. It also helps to have the sibling do some of the home exercises with their OT kid sibling that I send, that really hits home that they are a part of something big and important.)

When the whole family feels they are a part of the betterment of this OT kid than by golly you've got a group effort and an OT kid that has the best chance at meeting those whole person goals. Does this make sense? When I say the whole child, this also includes the family. It also includes their feelings, fears, hopes, frustrations, etc., etc. I tackle all of it using a whole repertoire of mediums, which I will talk about a little later. Okay, back to brain-body mapping . . .

I want to quote the following to lead into this brain-body mapping stuff because its good and I found it at the beginning of the book I mentioned earlier:

When a reporter asked the famous biologist J.B.S. Haldane what his biological studies had taught him about God, Haldane replied, "The Creator, if He exists (don't get me started about God, J.B.S.!)*, must have an inordinate fondness for beetles since there are more species of beetle than any other group of living creatures." By the same token, a neurologist may conclude that God is a cartographer. He must have an inordinate fondness for maps, for*

everywhere you look in the brain maps abound. *–V.S.*
Ramachandran

I was unaware of the beetle population being so
huge and now I'm just a bit freaked out but the last part
of this caught my attention. As I continued reading the
book, I couldn't put it down because it brought
everything, I have always wondered about but could
never put my finger on, into clear perspective.
JACKPOT!

Think about your arm for a minute then move it
in a big circle, now the other arm. Stick your tongue out
as far as you can and rotate your head in big circles. Try
to really feel the movements and space around you as
you do all of these zany things I have asked of you. Feel
for a hot minute that space around you relative to your
own body . . . this invisible vast volume of space around
your entire body out to arm's length and fingertips, the
top of your head where your halo is and down to the tips
of your toes is what scientists are now calling your
'peripersonal space' and it's all part of you. You may be

thinking, "Um, the crazy southern OT has lost it, bless her heart."

At times, yes, I do lose it especially when I have been wondering about things I couldn't solve for years and years, and they finally get answered!

Your body has this mapping procedure that it does to itself and literally feels it owns this space around you and clothes us in it like a ghostly skin. No, this isn't voodoo, I promise. These maps that encode our physical bodies are connected directly, immediately, and personally to a map of every point in that space and also map out your potential to perform actions in that space. In other words, your 'self' does not end where your flesh does.

For example, if you are a good horse rider, your body maps are blended with your horse's body maps during that riding time. When you get it on with your significant other, your body maps and your significant other's body maps commingle in your mutual passion and if they don't, um, you should rethink that relationship, just a suggestion.

Okay, let me simplify this some because it's a bit weird, I know. Think about when you are using a fork and knife to eat a kick-butt steak dinner. As you are holding the knife and fork, they become a part of your peripersonal space so that means that your brain's perception and self-ness doesn't stop at your fingertips while holding these two things, it will actually extend all the way down to the tip of each utensil essentially now being a part of you as far as your brain is concerned.

Think about a baseball player. The same thing happens once that kid or person picks up and holds that bat, to their brain, the bat has become a part of the self or the whole of the person. Make sense?

Think about this . . . have you ever driven into a parking garage that appears to be low and you can't help but to duck because you kind of feel like it's going to hit your head/top of the car? What is actually happening is that your brain has enveloped the entire car you are in from bumper to bumper and top to bottom so your ducking is a result of your brain claiming the space around it.

It's also like those poor souls, <u>me</u> for example, who lose a bunch of weight but still 'feel' fat. I recently lost 42 pounds using the Weight Watchers program and my mind still feels that my body is fat. There has not been a completed re-mapping yet of the area that mapped out that I was chubby, it takes time for this adjustment and I often preach on about this to the sweet folks in my Weight Watchers meetings. Sometimes the re-mapping can take too long and the person goes right back to their old ways and gains it all back. I'm hoping with this knowledge I have discovered that I will be patient while my brain re-maps so I don't get chubby again. God willing!

So, there are a couple of questions that are being asked about the body's response to the peripersonal space that surrounds us and the brain claiming that space as a part of you.

1. Why do we duck down in our cars if we perceive a garage entrance is a bit low as I just mentioned?

2. Why do your kids get sucked into video games with total and utter abandon to where you can yell their name and they don't hear you?

An aside, this peripersonal space brings up another neat thing that scientists have discovered called mirror neurons. These are the neurons that are responsible for you yawning when you see someone else yawn or why dudes watching a movie where some other dude gets nailed in the junk, grabs his own junk, and have known to moan. Crazy, huh?!

This is such interesting information that you may have wondered about and now neuroscientists are starting to figure out some cool stuff from their studies.

"What, pray tell crazy OT lady, does this have to do with OT?" Well, these neuroscientists have discovered, because of the collective effort of our numerous, flexible, morphable body maps, that this is the very thing that gives rise to the solid-feeling subjective sense of 'me-ness' thus giving us the ability to comprehend and navigate the world around us. In other words, if someone asked you how you knew that your hand was yours, you'd know because of the inner workings of these brain maps and all of the other bits that play their role in the performance of our brain and body mapping. I'll stop there because it gets a bit nutty so I'll move on.

A fascinating aside about the brain, and a correction that was long believed to be true, was that the window for successful treatment of a kid became narrow or in some ignorant opinions, closed completely, the older they got. Not true.

Did you know that you are able to increase your IQ all through your life unless you have some sort of organic brain syndrome because that makes things a bit tricky? Did you also know that our brain retains plasticity (the brain's ability to adapt and change as a result of experience) throughout our lives, again, if there is an organic brain syndrome or brain damage of some sort, this may not be or at least not able to happen as easily. So, if your kid is 13 and you know something is just not quite right, call an OT, ST, or PT and get them looked at. That window is not shut!

Let me say this though, some things are very hard to change, as I have explained this to my parents. One of the things that I have run into is trying to change the handwriting or grip on a pencil in an older kid. For some reason, handwriting and grip get stuck pretty tight in the brain and are very hard to change. That's just my experience. There are a few other things that I have had a hard time changing, but I'll digress here for now.

For the folks that work in pediatric OT land, we get kids whose brain-body maps get laid down in a less than functional way, therefore, losing a strong brain-body connection and our job is to re-map/connect these areas of trouble. Many things add to the mis-mapping/connection and we have already talked about a lot of them. Retained reflexes are the biggest one once the child is out of the womb. Another issue that I see a lot is with the kids that get adopted as I have several adopted angels on my caseload. These kids have a beginning that most of the adopting parents have no idea what possibly could have looked like but they take a chance anyway. God bless these folks.

For example, I had an OT kid years ago, before I knew what I know now, and I really struggled to help him get the gains he and his family were hoping for. It wasn't until a while later that I found out he was chained to his crib for hours on end and would often sit in his own poo thus causing horrific diaper rash.

So, let's break this down a bit from a brain-body mapping/connection perspective:

1. His brain-body map was confined to the peripersonal space of his crib meaning; his brain embodied that crib with his poo in it to boot. A very poor mapping situation, wouldn't you say?

2. He only moved within the practically static/not much movement confines of that crib therefore not getting the dynamic input of full-bodied movement that he was capable of and needed. And I will say it again here: MOVEMENT=LEARNING! So, DO NOT TAKE AWAY RECESS FROM THESE KIDS! FIND SOMETHING ELSE, PLEASE PLEASE PLEASE! THEY NEED TO MOVE! NEED, NOT WANT!

3. His butt was always on fire from sitting in poo for hours on end, therefore, a map of pain associated with his butt was laid, which later translated to holding his poo because of the association.

4. His bath was a hose down in his crib with cold water so afterward his crib remained wet and cold. Can you even imagine?

I'll not go on because I'm getting choked up. So, you see that this kid's brain-body maps were laid down in a very dysfunctional and quite sad and horrible way and also caused a huge disconnect between his brain and body, which I'll explain in a bit.

When I got him, he had retained reflexes, sensory processing issues big time, fear of closed spaces, extreme fear of being cold, holding his poo, and because his brain-body map was so messed up, if he ever got over-stimulated, he would violently gouge at the skin all over his sweet little self. His brain-body map of 'self' did not give him the sense of self-preservation or self-protection because of how poorly it was laid out and disconnected so he'd gouge the stew out of his face, his arms, and his legs. It was a nightmare. I wish I knew how he was doing but his family moved away at one point so I don't know. I pray for him even now, 15 years later.

Let me touch on my belief of why people kill or hurt themselves, just my opinion based on my OT knowledge. Our inherent human selves are supposed to be wired in a way so that we have a strong need to preserve ourselves, aka stay alive. For those folks who hurt or kill themselves, I think there is an addition to their depression and that's a huge brain-body disconnect plus poor brain-body mapping. This is just my take, so don't go trying to prove me wrong because I might be, I'm just throwing this out there for you to think about.

So, when I get a new OT kid, I look at the things that each kid is dealing with and I have to be fully aware of how that brain-body map was laid out and what their brain-body connection looks like. Here's where my job gets really really fun!

Have you ever heard of an XBOX 360 Kinect? Well, I have one and we use it a lot in conjunction with a bunch of other things with the kids on my caseload to aid in brain-body remapping/connection and it is working like a dream!

When I see a new OT kid that requires this type of treatment and I then introduce the Kinect, everyone looks at me like I've lost my mind but hear me out. First, I am not a big fan of static video games or playing on their phones for hours on end. It is not good for the kid's eyes because it causes near-sightedness (not being able to see things far away), screws up posture hence all the 'slumpy' children wandering around, and the flashing pictures stir up that Reticular Activating System (RAS) I spoke about earlier. TV has flashing pictures too so too much TV or video gaming especially before bed will mess up your sleep/wake cycle, therefore, causing a domino effect in your kid. They can't sleep well, therefore they may appear as if they have ADHD because they are actively trying to keep themselves awake during the day so they go to the extreme. They get misdiagnosed and then put on meds, but the real issue may be the video games or TV or on their cell phones right before bed. Everything in moderation!

I'd say video games or TV for NO more than 1-3 hours per day max, as for the cell phones, less is best but I know that is hard because being plugged in is a part of many of our careers, and our kid's social life, but do try to unplug when you can.

Break it up if you can and DO NOT LET THEM PLAY OR WATCH TV FOR AT LEAST 30-45 MINUTES BEFORE BED! You can kick me later but I know what I speak of! You to adults or you may not sleep well and we all need our healing sleep, believe me. That blue light stuff they talk about coming from electronics affects the levels of the sleep-inducing hormone melatonin in addition to the RAS I just spoke about. And some of you may say, "Well, there's always melatonin pills." Well, yes, and they may work for a time but if you take them for too long, your body will stop producing its own melatonin which is not a good thing!!! You'll be a mess if this happens.

Now answer me this, if you were riding your bike and you looked down to see what you could see while doing this, you'd be able to see your legs as they went up and down, your arms/hands holding on to the handlebars, and really only the scenery around you, right? Now, if your mom was watching you ride your bike, what is she seeing? Well, she is seeing EVERYTHING, but you can't because your eyeballs are in your head and they can't float out and away from your body to get the perspective that your mom has, right? And if you could do that then you might be possessed and your mom would pass out at the sight of your eyeballs exiting your head. Ew!

This is where that Kinect comes in. This super awesome system allows these kids to see what their body is doing, in other words, they get to be 'mom' seeing them on that bike for a bit because this Kinect system allows them to direct the body movements of the avatar in the games that I have them play.

One of my favorite games I use with the OT kids is the 'Adventure' game that came with my system. They get to see themselves stand in a raft and go down these rapids while shifting side to side to avoid these big poles in the water or they can jump up on the higher rocks and get more coins. My TV is big so the experience is even better. The other game I love on this disc is 'Reflex Ridge.' In this game, they are riding on an oversized skateboard, we'll say, and there are obstacles in front of them as they ride along that they have to duck, jump, and move to the side to avoid. Also, there are coin formations in different shapes that present themselves in front of them as they ride along, and in order to get all of the coins in the formation, they have to position their body into the shape they see, like a Y for example, so they'd put their feet together and they'd complete the Y with their arms above their heads in a V shape, thus getting every coin. This is a great game for many reasons but the spatial awareness input is awesome.

Why is this so cool? Well, think about it, they get to see their body move from an outside perspective and it is at this point the brain gets feedback it didn't have before and can start making corrections. It's also a lot of fun and you don't die in the games so I like that part too. This Kinect and the various other games that came with it plus, what I have purchased from Amazon, have a ton of the good things I would want to help my OT kid and their brain-body re-mapping/connection: vestibular input, visual input, proprioceptive input, timing, sequencing, attention to task, position in space, and a huge collected amount of feedback that the brain gets to help with the re-mapping/connection I've been talking about again, in a fun way. I've seen some cool stuff since

I have added this piece. I kid you not! Thanks, XBOX 360 KINECT!!!

One thing I get asked is wouldn't playing in front of a mirror give the same feedback? The answer is no, though I use mirrors for other reasons, which I will get to in the next paragraph, actually. Mirrors don't do what the Kinect does to the brain, however, they are very useful tools.

An aside, I have used this seeing-oneself-from-the-outside process throughout my career but it wasn't until now that I FULLY understood. When a parent is trying to teach a new skill to their childlike putting a shirt on, for example, I tell them to do it in front of a mirror because that way, the child can use their strongest sense to aid in learning what their body is doing and what is expected of them in order to get that shirt on. Make sense? This holds true for any new skill you want them to learn and parents, you can do this too. It helps to 'see' what your body is doing in order to learn a bit easier.

In conclusion, brain-body mapping starts in the womb at the brain stem level. The brain is one big map that gets more and more complex as life aids in the weaving. Sometimes there are bits to the map that don't develop fully or exactly as we would like to see, hence the re-mapping/connection OT's/therapists do.

It has been discovered that our brain encompasses the space around us coined our peripersonal space, which is like a ghostly skin we can't see but the brain is acutely aware of it like we talked about earlier. In order to tap into that re-mapping/connection, I have added the XBOX 360 Kinect to my repertoire of treatment. It's fun and the OT kids love it and don't even realize they are working their brain and body. There is a lot more on this subject of brain-body mapping/connection but I wanted you to have the meat, not that nasty garnish. Eck!

The Importance of Good Developmental Vision

I have many parents who have taken their child to an ophthalmologist or an optometrist and say, "Oh, the doc said their vision is good." This type of exam only evaluates visual acuity, the need for glasses, and eye health. There is a whole lot more to vision.

First of all, let's talk about the differences between the aforementioned eye people, shall we?

An ophthalmologist is an M.D. who has a lot more training/schooling and not only does the physical exam to see if you can see far and near, tests for glaucoma, and can prescribe glasses or contacts, this one handles eye disease and eye surgery.

The optometrist has a doctorate of optometry but they are not M.D.'S. They do all the things I just mentioned except for eye surgery.

A 'developmental' visual exam goes well beyond 20/20 and healthy eyes to assess a wide range of visual skills that are important for attention, learning, and reading.

Before I go on, I need to thank a man that doesn't even know me for his awesome sauce website of information that I always refer to when I have a child with what I believe are developmental eye issues. His name is Dr. Michael Gallaway, O.D. and he is a Pediatric Optometrist and offers Vision Therapy as well at his place in New Jersey. This guy is on it and I'm so happy to have found his website. Check out his website for checklists and questionnaires of what to look for with regard to your child's developmental vision. His website is www.drgallaway.com.

There are a lot of 'parts' to vision and it is imperative for school success and life success too, that those parts are working correctly. Let's talk about some of those parts and what they mean.

-<u>Visual processing or visual perception</u> is our brain's ability to interpret and analyze information that comes into our eyeballs. This is what I work on in OT with a lot of kids so this one I understand quite well. This 'part' is very important for letter and number recognition, reading and math skills, handwriting, the ability to copy work from the board onto their paper accurately, and to be able to organize schoolwork. Visual perceptual issues can arise in the following areas:

*<u>Visual form perception</u>-the ability to detect likes and differences in shapes, letters, numbers, and words.

*<u>Visual memory</u>-the ability to recall what you saw.

*<u>Directionality</u>-the ability to know your left from your right and up from down; this one is very important for reading as we read from left to right.

*<u>Visual processing speed</u>-the ability to process visual input quickly and accurately.

*<u>Visual-motor integration</u>-this can also be called eye-hand coordination really, but this is our body's ability to

work with the eyes by interpreting what the eyes have seen and then producing a motor output or movement.

Some signs of visual perceptual issues are:

-Letter and/or number and/or word reversals

-Poor handwriting

-Has trouble completing tests or classwork

-Has trouble copying from the board onto his/her paper

-Poorly organized written work

-Poor memory of visual material like sight words

-Seems to be a better auditory learner

Some additional 'parts' to the eye orchestration are eye teaming, focusing, and tracking, in other words, the <u>physical</u> ability of the eyes not the perceptual ability.

*Eye teaming can also be called 'binocular vision'-this is the fancy Nancy way of saying the ability of the eyes working together in a precise and coordinated way. There are two types of eye teaming issues: Convergence insufficiency-the tendency of the eyes to turn out while reading or doing close-up work. The other one is convergence excess-the tendency of the eyes to turn in while reading or doing close-up work.

*Focusing-this is the adjustments our eye muscles/ciliary muscles make quickly and accurately for looking far away and looking near like adjusting the focus on a camera.

*Tracking-I see this one A LOT, especially if several of the reflexes are retained, specifically the ATNR. This is when the eyes move quickly, smoothly, and accurately from place to place and can also be called 'visual scanning.'

So, as you can see, there are a lot of layers, if you will, to the eyes, and I've left out a lot of the parsley and given you the meat. Of course, my advice is to find a

DEVELOPMENTAL eye doctor. You should also hear the buzzwords I have just written to know for sure. Being able to see near and far doesn't mean a darn thing if your eyes aren't working together.

I really don't feel as if I should write the next section but I want to make sure there is a full understanding of why you have to be able to see and why all of your eye parts have to work.

Well, it'll affect reading and writing . . . so school work, basically. It can also be misdiagnosed as dyslexia or ADHD believe it or not. There are some folks out there that think visual issues <u>cause</u> dyslexia. Not so! Dyslexics, like myself, have trouble attaching sounds to letters and blend the sounds into words so it's 'phonetic,' not visual.

Also, visual problems don't cause ADHD but if your child is having trouble with his/her vision, they will look distracted during close up work by looking away (taking an eye break they don't even know they need but they know it helps), avoiding reading, or becoming fidgety from eye fatigue.

Now, the developmental eye doc I use here in Alabama likes for the kids to be at least 5 years old as it is easier to assess them. She also has a fabulous vision therapist that I refer to often because folks, I can do a lot as an OT, but I can't do it all.

For example, I don't do feeding therapy and I don't do certain types of vision therapy because it's a specialty that needs years of training. That's not to say I don't do any feeding therapy work, I do, with the reflex integrating exercises such as the one for the Rooting Reflex because this integration will help with feeding. I do work on visual perceptual skills, visual tracking, visual-motor skills, and convergence but if what I am doing is not getting the results my OT kid needs, I recommend vision therapy hands down as well as a feeding specialist.

There is a website I frequent called 'Eye Can Learn' and these folks have some nice eye exercises for tracking, visual perception, and a few more areas. My unbeknownst to him bestie Dr. Gallaway also has a tab with some games/exercises for the vision too. Again, his website is www.drgallaway.com.

Therapeutic Listening

Let me level with you on this program, I took this class out of complete and utter disrespect of the subject matter thinking it would be a knee slapper and a kick in the pants for something like this to actually work plus I needed the continuing education units to keep my license. Well, I was wrong, very wrong.

First, let's hash out what listening is. Listening is the ability and process of detecting sound, organizing those sounds, and integrating them for the blending of information from all of the other senses for functional and protective use. Listening is both conscious and unconscious. Unless you are deaf, you are constantly monitoring your auditory environment for the need to orient, locate, and select what you will do with the sounds we have tuned into. Listening is essential for survival in some cases. People that are deaf, on the other hand, count on vibrations, which is quite cool in my opinion, so they have their own way.

Let me try and give you the meat and not the parsley when I say that the vestibular system, or what I have loosely coined the 3-ring circus, is the system that lets your brain know where your head is in space. This system has a large part in the improvement of many sensory integration issues. Here's the cool thing about the vestibular system, it is married, if you will, to the auditory system (you may have heard it generally called the cochlea although it has two friends named utricle and saccule, just as important), which kind of makes sense since it's also located in the ear. If you were to look at this little organ, there is no clear-cut boundary between the two.

Now, why is this so cool? Well, neurologically speaking, these two systems function in much the same manner with hair-like receptors moving in a fluid-filled canal. They also share a single cranial nerve, which is key to the success of Therapeutic Listening (TL). This shared nerve sends information to the brainstem (where the reflexes just so happen to hang out, if you remember) and then crosses paths and exchanges more information with each other every step of the way. Wouldn't it be nice if all marriages were like this?!

To get all fancy Nancy on you, this system, or marriage for those of you that this makes sense to, is called the vestibular-cochlear system. Now, if you really want to see the coolest video around that shows you what I'm talking about, please look this video up on YouTube, it is super cool!!!

https://youtu.be/PeTriGTENoc

Once you've seen this video then what I am about to talk about will really make more sense.

Alright, because the vestibular-cochlear system is designed in the way that it is (filled with little hair-like structures with fluid in the canal with them as well as these little crystals called otoliths that get moved around by sound waves coming in thus, scooting those little crystals across the hair giving loads of input to the vestibular system and the brain) something really cool happens in the brain. Where this all fires off in the brain is right next to the speech center. That's why OTs and STs will sometimes co-treat together. The OT will rile up that vestibular system (by swinging and spinning, for example), and sometimes as it is firing in the brain, there is a 'spill,' if you will, into the surrounding brain tissue thus tickling the speech center, which greatly helps out the child's speech during his/her session. It's really cool!

So, Therapeutic Listening was pioneered by Sheila Frick, also an OT and she must have thought, "Well, I'll be. I can use this listening stuff through sound waves that are modified to tickle those hairs a certain way and fire off just splendidly in the brain." She may have not thought that exactly but you get the gist. She's awesome and I stand corrected Sheila, so, please forgive me. You rock sister, with your Therapeutic Listening and all!

Okay, here is some more meat on this subject. TL has allowed therapists to add to or expand the world of sensory integration. It is a genius auditory intervention that uses a series of organized sound patterns inherent in music to affect all areas of the nervous system. If you couple your sensory integration activities with TL some really neat things happen thus, speeding up some of the gains that your OT kid will get, such as:

-Attention

-More organized behavior

-Self-regulation

-Postural control

-Bilateral coordination

-Praxis (the neurological process by which cognition directs motor action)

-Fine motor control

-Oral motor/articulation

-Social skills

-Communication

-Visual motor integration

I know I thought, "Are you freaking kidding me crazy Sheila lady," but no, no she isn't because this stuff works! She's another of my besties that are unaware they are on my list.

I use this Therapeutic Listening program proudly in my clinic with many of my OT kids and I have seen great things. Like a child who wasn't talking at all and with some OT magic in the clinic, reflex integrating, and this TL program, the boy is talking!

If you are interested in learning more about this further, please visit Sheila's website: www.vitalsounds.com. You can also check out the folks at Advanced Brain Technologies at www.advancedbrain.com. This is another good resource doing a similar therapy.

The Brushing and Joint Compression Protocol

I learned this protocol ages ago and must give credit for the creation of this program to a gal named Patricia Wilbarger, M.Ed., ORT, FAOTA.

This program was designed by Patricia to help the brain organize itself, basically. Our skin is the largest organ of the body followed by the muscles and skeletal systems, which are connected by our nervous system and the brain is the boss of it all. So, given this, Patty (can I call you Patty?) came up with a technique that involves one of those surgical brushes brushed across the skin in a certain way on certain body parts followed by joint compressions or gently pushing the joint into itself.

When I was taught this procedure years ago, I only used it if a child had a pretty rough relationship with their skin meaning, they did not like touch, they hated tags, they would only wear certain types of clothing, etc. You may have also heard this being called 'tactile defensiveness.'

I use this on a regular basis now, in addition to using it with tactile issues, if I see a disconnect in a child from their peripersonal space, trouble with spatial awareness in general, a brain-body mapping issues, retained reflexes, and to help calm them and connect with their parent. I love this program and I don't always do all of it. For example, I am currently treating my own husband who has a retained Fear Paralysis, Moro, and Spinal Galant, as I have mentioned. I use brushing <u>only</u> with him and not the joint compression because I'm after a 'calm state' for him.

If you remember from earlier, I mentioned that the Fear Paralysis and Moro put the body in a constant state of the feeling of fight or flight and that's horrible if you think about it, always being edgy waiting for something to scare the stew out of you and he's jumpy, very jumpy and I'm so glad I helped him figure it out.

I had him fill out that checklist of retained reflexes and he was shocked at the insight he gained from this. It also taught me a lot about him and I love him even more if that's even humanly possible.

So, for him, I do a combo. Each morning, afternoon, and evening I have him lay on the bed and I brush both arms front and back including the hands, not the under pits, that's too tickly, then his legs and feet top and bottom, but not his inner thigh, also too tickly, then his back. I spend a long time with him, especially his back because of that retained Spinal Galant he's got. He also does his reflex integrating exercises for the Fear Paralysis, Moro, and the Spinal Galant once a day, twice if we can swing it. I do them with him because of my retained Moro and Spinal Galant and we giggle at each other as we are doing them but we are bonding in a way that I doubt many folks have, therapeutically. Crazy life.

I've also added the cold laser therapy I mentioned earlier and we are seeing good things happening.

Okay, so this program is usually followed by joint compressions, or pushing the joint into itself but not violently, is the best way to describe it. So, let's say you are giving your child joint compressions into their shoulder, you would hold your child's elbow with one hand and your other hand would sit on top of their shoulder otherwise, if you push up into the shoulder joint without that stabilizing hand on the top of the shoulder, you'd just push their shoulder into their ear. You need counter pressure to activate the proprioceptive receptors in the joints and muscle bellies. Does that make sense? You can YouTube this program to get the feel of what I am talking about if it doesn't make sense.

Anyway, this program is a good one and I have seen good things out of it too. I don't always use it in the way that it was designed but I have reasoned that sometimes you don't have to do everything exactly; you need to tweak it for your OT kid's and in my case your husband's purposes. Lord knows I've bent and tweaked quite a lot of 'techniques/protocols' over the years with great results too because I believe in listening to my gut and heart as a therapist and human being.

This technique needs to be taught to you from an OT, PT, or ST who has been trained in it because if you goof up and accidentally brush the neck or the belly, bad reactions can happen like vomiting, a disturbance in blood flow, or even seizures. Not kidding!

This technique can be Googled for more information if you want the parsley; I'm just the meat girl, no garnish, please.

Brain Beat

Brain what? Yes, the beating of the brain! Naw, just kidding. Let me back up some so you can get the full appreciation of why this is an awesome treatment option.

So, 100 years ago, there was really no way to treat or at least attempt to treat ADD and ADHD other than humming pills at it, which has become the way with a lot of doctors when it comes to children. Again, I call this lazy doctoring, hands down. There is a deeper reason why kids have what they have and yes, I'll say it again, go back to that brainstem, darn it, because that's where a lot of it is coming from. Not all of it, but I'll bet it has a hand in whatever you are seeing. Stop chucking pills at the kids, it's wrong! Not to mention the secondary side effects on top of the issue.

Have you ever seen those commercials for some new drug and the side effects seem to outweigh the actual issue at hand? My family and I always get a charge out of the announcer saying, "Side effects might include death, dismemberment, alienism, zombie-type behavior, removal of all of your flesh, headlessness, eyeball loss, etc., etc." You get my point. Why would I want to fix one thing and then have to take on 22 other things to make this pill fit me?

Okay, back to Brain Beat. So, nothing much to treat attention issues with other than the slinging of a pill in your child's mouth. My mom refused to medicate me, as I said before, and put me in every sport she could to wear me out. It still didn't fully help my issue though.

Several years ago, all of a sudden, a treatment came out that utilized a metronome beat with motor movement to keep up with that beat, and lo and behold, in addition to helping kids with ADD and ADHD, it was also helping other things like autism, dyslexia, SPD, general learning disabilities, folks recovering from a stroke, and many more areas. I was floored and in the only way I know how to behave when something genius is discovered, I read everything I could and eventually became certified in Interactive Metronome Therapy.

If I wanted, I could actually have an extra set of 'letters' behind my name and it would be this: IMC, but I don't roll that way. Who cares how many letters are behind your name because most people have no idea what it stands for anyway and it doesn't make you a better medical person. Especially if your bedside manner stinks or you just throw pills at people because you are too lazy to get to the root of the issue. Good thing you have folks like OTs, PTs, STs, etc. who are willing to get into the trenches and figure it out without meds.

The Interactive Metronome Therapy folks say that rhythm and timing are at the heart of all human abilities. What that means in girlfriend terms is our ability to attend and focus, to take notes while the teacher is giving instruction, keeping up with the conversation in a group of friends, reading and attaching meaning to written words, jumping, skipping, riding a bike, and learning and retaining new information. For folks with developmental or acquired issues (like a head injury from a car accident, for example), their timing and rhythm are very much affected and just adds to their difficulties.

An aside . . . I got the honor and privilege years ago to work with an 18-year-old up-and-coming actor on his timing. He had landed a role in that first Percy Jackson movie and can be seen in the high school at his locker scene. He exchanges a line with Percy but the problem with his delivery was timing. His coach said, "Find an OT and get hooked up with this metronome treatment so you can deliver your line properly and timely before you come to Hollywood and we start shooting."

Guess what, I got to hang out with him and work on his timing using, at that time, the Interactive Metronome Therapy and he got a lot better, flew out, did his movie, and did awesomely. I love this little dude and loved getting to know him and his mother. Not sure what he has gone onto do after the Percy Jackson gig but I'll bet it's great!

The Interactive Metronome folks describe their program as "a brain-based, multi-disciplinary assessment and treatment tool that has been shown, in clinical research, to improve the neurological functions of motor planning, sequencing, timing, and attention."

Layman's terms for this simply means your ability and the fluidity of the way you move through life like reaching out for a glass of water, walking, talking in a shared conversation without interrupting, or arranging words in a sentence so what you are saying makes sense. Hence, my sweet actor dude not interrupting Percy when it was time for his line or delivering it too late.

The Interactive Metronome folks did all the research and can back up all of what they claim with well-documented research and I thank them for this.

One day, one of my awesome sauce counselor friends texted me this spin-off of the Interactive

Metronome Therapy I was using and I liked it a lot plus, the lay folk could buy it for use at home, as it was very user friendly and affordable. Most of my OT kids prefer to come and work on it with me absolutely refusing to do it at home as they say, "It's not the same mom. I have to be with Ms. Sharon." Awww! Brain Beat is awesome and although 'Nigel' the avatar drives me a bit batty, as I hear him talk all day long, bless him, he's sweet and I actually have one little girl who will kiss the computer screen and tells me that Nigel is her boyfriend because he is so cute. LOL!

During one of my Brain Beat or Interactive Metronome sessions with the kids, here's what happens, the child can choose from a tapper (looks like a game show buzzer), a quiet tapper (flat with a yellow circle in the middle and doesn't click like the tapper), or a hand clapper that Velcro's around with the switch in the palm of their hand. The goal is to clap exactly on the beat or 'cowbell,' as the kids like to call it. The screen gives them colored feedback, in other words, green is awesome, yellow is okay, and red means you've got to focus a bit better. The boxes let them know if they are hitting too late or too early and there is a number that comes up when each box is lit up. The number is the average milliseconds they are off of the beat. The lower the number the better and zero is perfect, meaning you were dead on the beat. This is hard to do and the kids and I have established that Jesus could maybe swing all zeros, as He is perfect. Oh, these kids!

There are also different worlds to conquer like the jellyfish world, robo-dog world, a bug-eating frog world, and many more in Brain Beat.

Also, the kids can also level up from silver to gold to platinum and if their millisecond score is low enough, THE RHYTHM MASTER! If you are The Rhythm Master, you are royalty in my OT kid's eyes. I have only had 3 in all my years but I see a couple of my current OT kids making it and I'm really thrilled for them. Their picture gets put on the wall and it's a big deal. Also, as they level up, their name is added next to the medal they leveled up to plus they get a medal necklace to take home and show their families. This is very exciting for them.

You are encouraged to stand up as that makes the kids more dynamic and their brain is turned on a bit more. I'll tell you; the kids figure out 'their own way' and I allow that because I'd rather have them choosing their own way as they are more successful at this program. It is being absorbed no matter what and they're more apt to participate if <u>they</u> have the choice. I don't do power struggles in OT as it adds resistance. My take is as long as I am helping them meet their goals, I'll dance the dance I have to; however, I have a lot of tricks up my sleeve.

During Brain Beat, I may do hand over hand to help them clap or tap as needed especially if I see a kid getting frustrated or ticked off. Plus, that skin-to-skin contact is another really important element to being a therapist. Now, I'm not saying get all weird with it but our society has blown 'touching' way out of proportion and I get it but it's time to chill out. The life scale gets tipped so far sometimes that it borders idiotic and ridiculous. Wouldn't you agree?

I hug, I hold hands, I let the kids sit on my lap (they love this the most for some reason), and I kiss the tops of their little sweet halo heads a lot, they need this, they really do. They just need to know that they are 'in', that they belong, and they matter.

So, look Brain Beat up at www.brainbeat.com. I use this with almost all of the kids each time I see them and the way I tell them how it works is this, "Have you ever had a tangle in your hair after you went swimming or got out of the shower? Yes? Well, it's kind of a pain to get out, isn't it? So, you get a comb and gently, carefully, and slowly work on that tangle until it's free, right? Well, think of Brain Beat as the comb working that tangle out slowly but surely. Your brain has all these things called synapses that bridge places all over your brain and sometimes if you are having trouble with your attention or reading or math what that means is those synapses are running tangled-like instead of smoothly as they should be. Cue the Brain Beat comb to the rescue to help these synapses untangle and run smoothly." They get this and I'll bet you do too now.

Some therapists will torture a child for the full 30 minutes of a session (I actually see kids 45 minutes to an hour each session, 30 minutes IS NOT ENOUGH in my opinion) using either Interactive Metronome or Brain Beat. This is a tool, and I'll bet a dime to a dollar you couldn't build a whole house with just a hammer, right? You have to use a myriad of tools to do that with but to each their own. I will spend about 10 minutes or so on this unless they are rocking it, and then we move on because what have I said before? MOVEMENT=LEARNING and you can't stay at a still activity for too long or you lose brain and body momentum.

Brain Beat has really worked wonders in many of these kids, not all of them though because we are all wired differently and different things work with different people. Check it out or ask your therapist about it if they aren't already using it.

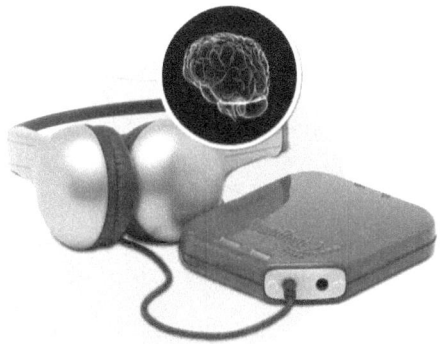

Yoga

When I used to hear the word 'yoga' I used to picture that chubby little Buddha dude and a bunch of crazy people contorting their bodies into unthinkable positions with weird incense burning and a lot of 'Om-ing.'

Well, I'm very wrong of course, and now use yoga as part of my treatment with the OT kids on my caseload and I used to teach Saturday mornings too, but I have gotten way too busy and had to take a break, unfortunately. I'd teach three different kid yoga classes for kids who were not necessarily on my caseload. It was a blast and I got to do it my way so what that means is we had 'boot camp' yoga sessions for my older boys, 'obstacle course' yoga with my girls, and yoga stories where we went into the ocean to save 'Nemo' who was stuck in a treasure chest or we flew to Africa and checked out the animals there. You can go nuts with kid yoga and I want to thank my awesome sauce instructor out of

England who gave me the greatest yoga video critique I could have ever asked for therefore getting my certification as a kid yoga instructor.

Her name is Jamie Amor and her website is www.cosmickids.com. She is the greatest teacher and one of the nicest people on the planet plus, she made learning yoga loads of fun.

An aside, I did take Pilates for years because it sounded more sophisticated than yoga when I was ignorant, and I loved it. It made me strong, flexible, confident, and I felt capable of anything. My back stopped hurting, I had definition in my arms, and I felt awesome after each class. Life got in the way and I haven't been able to go as much as I'd like but that is a goal I don't want to lose track of. My point is, I use Pilates in my OT sessions as well and it is good for the kids too.

Why kid's yoga? Well, one of the things that I have seen increasing in children is the lack of a calm self, poor posture, poor core strength, an altered sense of self, and poor self-esteem. This really bothers me and I'm seeing it more and more. So, one day, I was messing around on Facebook and saw that a friend of mine was teaching adult yoga. I messaged her back and forth for a bit getting her take on yoga for kids and what she was seeing with yoga for adults. I was intrigued with what she had to say and then I ran across another friend teaching adult yoga and picked her brain a bit too.

One day, just for kicks, I thought I'd see what was involved in getting kid yoga certified, and then I found my new bestie Jamie and her Cosmic Kids website and was hooked. Jamie is the cutest woman and as I said, as sweet as can be. Her enthusiasm for what she does is very contagious.

In order to get certified, I had to complete all of the sections to the class, pass the tests, and then make a video of a class that I would teach, no kids were there but I pretended there were, and sent it to her.

Now, let me just tell you a bit about me. I am not a showy person, I do not like to be on video or in photos, and I know my limitations when it comes to photogenic-ness. I am not a photogenic specimen and that's okay. I've been on TV only once on the health section of the news and I'm surprised I made it through the interview, as I almost passed out. I have been asked back a lot but turn it down. I just can't, as it is not me.

Several months back a local magazine asked me for an interview about being a Pediatric OT and then asked when a good time to schedule 'the photo shoot' for the front cover. I almost wet my pants but I will say, although I felt like I was going to throw up during the 'shoot,' the pictures turned out surprisingly well and I got razzed from many of my friends but they agreed it was a great picture and the article was good too.

One of my silly sausage neighbors was walking his dog by my house the day after the magazine came out and caught me outside watering my plants and says this to me, "Oh, well, there she is in all of her glory! The magazine cover super-star and here's lowly me and my lowly dog wanting to walk past the house of the great

OT among us." Needless to say, I about fell out laughing and threw a piece of mulch at him yelling, "You are a big fat goober now cut it out, you are embarrassing the stew out of me!" He's a goober all right but a hoot and I love his wife, we go way back.

So, making this video for Jamie was soooooo far out of my comfort zone but I do it anyway because I really worked hard and wanted my certification. Within a week or two, Jamie got back to me via her own critique video and she made me blush all over again. She said that she couldn't help but laugh out loud at my southern drawl and all the 'y'all's' I'd say throughout my video. She said a bunch of other very sweet and wonderful things but the best thing she said was that I passed with flying colors and that she saw great things for me as a kid yoga instructor. I was honored in so many ways and proud that I overcame fears just for this one video. She did go onto say that I should make videos as she does on YouTube because kids would love them.

Soooo, despite my discomfort behind a camera and/or acting aka teaching yoga to a class that is not actually there, I'm thinking about making more kid yoga videos with an OT twist to them and putting them on YouTube. As of now, there is only one on there and it is the one I had to send in for critiquing by Jaime. I put it out there when I had to stop teaching yoga on Saturday mornings. My YouTube channel is titled 'Dragonfly Pediatric Therapy.' I am so out of my comfort zone but I realize that kids need this and I'm all about the kids plus, it's kind of like my own stand-up comedy act with yoga thrown in. My husband says I'm a big goofball and he's right, I am.

Kid yoga and the poses within the yoga classes are just a modified version of adult yoga and some of the poses are named differently like the frog, the crab, the flamingo, etc. to make it fun for the kids. I believe, hands down, that this is a very important piece to any practice and really, it would be great to do at home as there are loads of good kid yoga videos, especially Jamie's on Cosmic Kids Yoga on YouTube and maybe just maybe, you might check mine out someday. Kid yoga really helps all around but also with the following:

-Develop body awareness

-Learn how to use their bodies in a healthy way

-Manage stress through breathing, awareness, meditation, and healthy movement

-Build concentration

-Increase their confidence and positive self-image

-Feel part of a healthy, non-competitive group

-Increase core strength, which is important for all human beings

    If you can add yoga into your OT session that would be great but if not, I encourage you to find a class, your child will benefit greatly.

Hippotherapy or Equine Assisted Therapy

No, we don't use hippos in therapy and no equine isn't a crochet stitch that your great Aunt Edna is teaching the folks at the assisted living place she asked to move into. 'Hippo' is the Greek word for horse and the word 'equine' means a horse or any member of the horse family.

About 100 years ago, when I was a little girl, I discovered what a horse/pony was at the age of 5 when I got the chance to ride on one at the Illinois State Fair round and round in a circle. I later began watching Western shows with my dad and found myself getting very upset if one of the horses got hurt. Never mind the cowboy that just got thrown off and hit his head on a rock and is probably dead, just don't hurt the horses! I would ask for horse books for my birthday and check them out a lot at the library as much as I could.

I was obsessed with horses and wanted one so bad, it hurt and no Ma, a baby bunny from the Easter bunny isn't a horse and you know it, it's cute and all but it isn't a horse. Thank you anyway. Lol, love you Ma . . . you too Dad!!

An aside, my mom wanted a pony from the time she was a child too. It never happened for her either but my two sisters and I like to give her cards and stuffed animals that are ponies just to mess with her. My mom rocks and she has been a huge influence on me, thus helping to mold me into the insane person I have become. I am very blessed and thankful.

Moving on . . . so for Christmas every year, I would get a horse statue/figure made out of plastic or glass and then later a barn to keep all of them in, not the glass ones of course. These horses were as precious as gold to me and I took very good care of them.

Later on, we discovered that there was a horse next to my dad and his brother's farm that the neighbor didn't really take care of too well. We didn't live on the farm, we just hung out and did farm stuff like hayrides, shooting, getting lost, fishing, my dad and his brothers hunted, etc., but no, no horse of our own, boo! Even though we had the land, we just didn't have the money or the time!

My sisters, cousins, and I loved this horse to bits and would bring him carrots every time we came to the farm, which was a lot. Eventually, I got brave, climbed the fence, and began riding 'Gold Dust' bareback around the next-door farmer's land. It was awesome and I used to pretend that Gold Dust was my horse. Unfortunately, this make-believe-it-was-my-horse lasted a short time because we moved from Illinois, when I was 13, to Alabama, as I mentioned earlier.

My love of horses has always been there. I love the way they look with their long strong necks and their flowing main and tail when they run, plus they just look so proud, so aware of their power and grace. Yes, I am in love way too deep with something I didn't think I'd ever own or be around, but alas, the heart wants what it wants.

After I graduated from OT school, I heard about this therapy called Hippotherapy and yes, at first, I thought, "What an absolutely bizarre treatment using Hippos. Wouldn't the kids get killed?" Obviously, I needed to do research and in the way that I always work, I bought every book and took every class, except I didn't get certified because, at this point, I didn't know of anyone looking to team up with me to do this type therapy using horses. I sadly and reluctantly put it on the back burner and I thought, "It'll never happen, it's not meant to be, Sharon, hang it up, sister."

So, I did and moved onto some of the other things that I have mentioned thus far but I'm not done introducing you to The Dragonfly Approach, nope there are more things to tell you and we will get there.

Several months ago, I ran into a colleague, who I have worked with here and there over the years, at the Autism Walk and like God always does, He had me run

into her on purpose, and here's what happily bloomed . .
.

My friend/colleague introduced me to her PATH certified horse friend, who is now my partner in my new addition to what I have to offer from my repertoire of treatment that I believe with all my heart is really good stuff!

Now, my partner is one of the coolest, smartest, calls-it-like- she-sees-it chicks around, and she is God-given to me. I'll call her the 'Crazy Cadillac Lady,' (C.C.L.) she gets that because of something I said about her horse, "I didn't know, C.C.L., okay?!" She is also PATH certified, which is a big deal in the horse world.

According to the PATH International website, this certification means: The "Professional Association of Therapeutic Horsemanship International, which is a federally registered 501 (c3) nonprofit formed in 1969 as the North American Riding for the Handicapped Association to promote equine-assisted activities and therapies (EAAT) for individuals with special needs." It's impressive, she's impressive, and I'm so thankful for her.

C.C.L. and I are 'one-woman' shows and in our Hippotherapy, we focus on quality, not quantity. She and I are alike in that we both possess a wide variety of knowledge and we are absolutely addicted to learning more. She trains and competes her own horses on a regular basis and teaches a few select students riding lessons. C.C.L. has a strong background in classical dressage and emphasizes safety and the well-being of the horse and rider while promoting independence using the power of the horse. (Her words, not mine. Told you she was smart.)

I get asked a lot about what the difference is between Hippotherapy and Therapeutic Riding, please see the picture below that I borrowed from the Granit State Carriage Association. They nailed the differences perfectly. All of the differences aside though, being around a majestic horse is therapeutic in and of itself, even if you don't get on one. There's just something about being in their presence, watching them, petting them, and giving them a carrot now and again. It settles a person's soul, it really does.

Hippotherapy	Therapeutic Riding
Physical, Occupational or Speech Therapy. Every step and movement of the horse is a treatment tool.	Adapted recreational horseback riding lessons.
Hippotherapy is NOT a horseback riding lesson. It is physical, occupational or speech therapy which is prescribed by a physician and delivered by a team that includes a licensed therapist.	Therapeutic riding is a recreational horseback riding lesson adapted to individuals with disabilities.
Hippotherapy is completed by a professional therapist in conjunction with a professional horse handler and a specially screened and trained therapy horse.	Therapeutic riding is completed by a professional riding instructor in conjunction with volunteers.
Direct hands-on participation by the therapist at all times.	The individual is often taught riding lessons in a group format which runs in sessions. The instructors must respond to the group as a whole.
The horse's movement is essential to assist in meeting therapy goals.	There is occasional hands-on assistance by the riding instructor and/or volunteers, but the instructor usually teaches from the center of the arena.
The goal of hippotherapy is for professional treatment to improve neurological functioning in cognition, body movement, organization and attention levels.	Horses used for therapeutic riding instruction have been screened to make sure they have the appropriate temperament for this job.
Hippotherapy is a one-on-one treatment and generally occurs year round until the client meets discharge criteria.	In therapeutic riding, the emphasis is on proper riding position and rein skills, not functional therapeutic goals.
In hippotherapy, the treating therapist continually assesses and modifies therapy based on the client's responses.	Because therapeutic riding is an adaptive sport, NOT therapy, is it not covered by insurance.
Insurance should pay for physical, occupational or speech therapy in which hippotherapy is used.	

My partner can teach Therapeutic Riding Lessons too but at this time, she is mostly focusing on Hippotherapy with me and I'm so honored.

Tangent alert . . . Check out my cute logo for Hippotherapy. I just love it! I used my buddy on Fiverr to help me design all of my logos and he nails it every time. Love you, Fiverr Edi! If you like his work, you can find him at https://instagram.com/happysketchy/. He is very good at what he does!

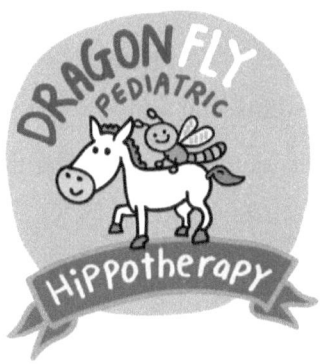

There are many benefits to doing OT with horses and I'll list a few of them:

-Reducing muscle tone seen in spasticity

-Improves attention and postural control

-Decreases sensory defensiveness

-Helps with fine-motor skills when the child uses the tack supplies or helps with grooming the horse

-Sensory integration

-Gross-motor skills

-The rhythmic movements of the horse help to facilitate the psychological systems that support speech and language skills as well as follows along the lines of a treatment I use called "The Rhythmic Movement Method" (see the Appendix for this awesome book)

-Overall brain-body organization

-Builds confidence

-Helps with spatial awareness

-And loads more but I'll stop there otherwise this book will be 400 pages long, yes, there are tons more benefits!

Now, I realize having this piece to your practice or expecting your therapist to provide this piece is a lot, but I am blessed and honored to be able to offer this to my OT kids along with the awesome input from my partner, C.C.L. However, if you know of a program in your area, go, as you will not be disappointed in all the good things it can do for your child.

I can't very well leave out my other horse friend, Amy, as she is my bestie for real and was the start of teaching me all about horses in the real-life setting and not from books or videos.

She is a chick that was born on a horse and when I go to the 'barn' with her to groom, ride, and be around what I love, she comes to life and it's really cool to see. She is teaching me Western riding and I love the laid-back tone of this type of riding. She is also a decorated horsewoman herself and her riding of choice in horse shows at the moment is dressage. I love you awesome sauce, Amy. You provide therapy for my soul when you let me tag along to the barn and I thank you from the bottom of my 'hippo-loving heart.'

A bit of warning about Hippotherapy, there are contraindications and they have to be adhered to for the safety of everyone involved, horse included. Some of them are:

-Spinal fusion/fixation

-Spinal instabilities/Abnormalities

-Osteoporosis

-Hydrocephalus/Shunt

-Seizures

-Dangerous to self or others

-Heart conditions

-Recent surgeries

-Indwelling catheters

Again, these are just some, and if you are interested in knowing all of them you can look at the PATH website: www.pathintl.org.

One of the things that I have been learning on my Hippotherapy journey is that the horse is the therapist and I just guide. For example, just brushing a horse works on a ton of things like upper body range of motion, crossing the midline, hand strength, upper body strength for sure, etc. You don't necessarily have to do this grandiose crazy looking treatment during a Hippotherapy session. Sometimes you just have to let the child sit or ride slowly because this does something to them. Being up high on this large majestic animal, looking at the trees and the Earth around them, spending some time outside in the sun breathing clean oxygen, that's the therapy right there. Remember when I told you I treat the whole child? That very much includes mental health, confidence building, and appreciating their bodies in nature. Nature heals. It always has and it always will.

Recently, I realized a need for groundwork as some of the kids aren't ready or willing to get up on a horse and that is okay. So, I found a lovely lady named Kathi who runs a not-for-profit ranch called Happy Trails Therapeutic Riding Center. Boy, has she taught me some things about natural horsemanship in the short time I have known her. She is trained in the Parelli

Method and if you want more information on this, please go to the website: www.parelli.com.

Her facility is a licensed SpiritHorse Therapeutic Riding Center, which offers a research-based, award-winning curriculum originally designed for kids with autism but has since been modified for other disabilities. Kids with all sorts of challenges can benefit from being in the horse's presence as well as riding if they are interested. Her kids interact with the horses by grooming and then playing communication games with them. These activities help with physical health, self-confidence, and independence. Kathi's facility is a Therapeutic Riding Center and as of now, not a place to do Hippotherapy, but maybe someday.

Some of the benefits of her program are:

-Stretching of tight or spastic muscles

-Improvement of reflexes

-Strengthening muscles and core

-Increased mobility

-Increase range of motion

-Improved respiration, circulation, appetite, and digestion

-Improved mental health

I am so blessed and lucky to know these three women who have graced my life and practice with their presence and expertise.

Every once in a while, I am unable to carry out my Hippotherapy or Equine Assisted Therapy because I get so busy in the clinic so I send my kids/families to Happy Trails or Hope Horses, another therapeutic facility I found recently, here locally.

I also want to point out that therapy using horses is not just for kids. It is also for veterans of war. I have heard some of the neatest jaw-dropping stories from one of my other horse friends who runs a horse-assisted veterans' program near me. I am so proud that we have access to this in our area. Our veterans need and deserve this very helpful therapy.

Aquatic Therapy

As I mentioned at the beginning of this book, I was certified many years ago as an aquatic therapist but started out using it with adults and geriatric citizens early in my OT career. I loved it, they loved it, and it was very useful for many of my patients.

Another thing I set on the back burner (after I left my first job using aquatics) was the use of aquatics in my therapy all throughout my career until now, as I moved several times and had several jobs and none of them had a pool. However, God came to me and helped me find a way.

Have you ever been looking for your keys or your sunglasses and you look and look, growing more and more irritated because you are late already and that darn carpool line isn't getting any 'funner' the longer you delay? You get stabby; maybe you kick the dog dish over in your haste so now there's that to contend with later.

Then a weird-ish thing happens, your head starts to itch, you naturally reach up to scratch it, and lo and behold there are your 'missing' glasses right on top of your head.

Now, if it's me in this sunglass's situation, one of two things can occur:

1) I say loud cuss words at no one, although the dog thinks he's pooped somewhere again but he really doesn't remember. Maybe it just fell out of him so he goes scurrying off to hide under the bed because his crazy southern lady owner has lost her freaking mind again.

2) I laugh at myself and realize I have gotten strung out again with too much running through my mind, kind of like that dog chasing its tail.

The keys are an entirely different set of responses for me . . .

As I'm looking frantically for them, I notice that something has stuck me in my palm and as I look to inspect who or what dare stick me, yep, there are my keys in my freaking hand. Here's what I could possibly think:

1) I decide I've gone mad and really should seek help from a professional.

2) I need more sleep.

3) I need a car that doesn't need keys to start, just mind control would be awesome and appreciated.

4) Why am I looking for my keys anyway, I don't even have carpool today-I need professional help.

So, this is what happened to me with God who looked down at me, shook His head, and nudged me in the direction of approaching my parents who own a lovely pool, they are close to the clinic, and my OT kids need this. I had yet another 'duh' moment at why I hadn't thought of this before. I had a chat with my mom and dad and they said no problem just have them sign waivers. Easy peasy, um, thank God for the much-needed nudge. I can't tell you how many 'duh' moments I have every stinking hour it seems. You know most people have those 'a-ha' moments, well no, not me, mine are more like 'duh' moments. Sigh.

The aquatic therapy that I do is in about 3 feet of water with steps to access the pool. I don't have any OT kids on my current caseload that would need another way to get in because of a wheelchair, for example, but I'll get to that dilemma in a bit. I have every pool or bath toy imaginable and pretty much anything I do with the kids in the clinic, I can do in the pool. Such things as:

-Crossing the midline

-Eye-hand coordination

-Overall body strength

-Range of motion

-General body coordination

-Core strength

-Visual tracking

-Reflex integrating exercises

-Sensory integration work

-Yoga

-And a whole lot more

Some unique things about water that you may not know, or maybe you do but are just modest, is that there is this property called hydrostatic pressure, which covers the kids in a blanket of deep relaxing pressure. It's like a "water hug.' Don't hugs just feel good anyway? If you haven't had a hug in a while, put this book down and go hug it out with someone right this minute. You need this!

When the hydrostatic pressure gives a water hug to the child's body, it gives the central nervous system some nice information like where the body is in space, for example. Other areas of improvement that you might see in your child who is doing aquatic therapy are better motor planning, self-regulation, speech, oral-motor control, strength, coordination, and endurance.

Again, I cannot stress the importance and the benefit of being outside in the sun and in the fresh air. Yes, the sun could give us skin cancer but with every bad, there is a good, right? That's how life works, it's not perfect, it's not always clean and organized, it doesn't always help you out when you've lost your glasses again, but life is a beautiful thing so get out of the house and get out there. Plus, research shows that there are undeniable benefits to being in the sun and breathing fresh air. Not to mention the gorgeous things God has given us. Enjoy the gifts because one day, you might not be able to. Life does have an expiration date after all.

The dilemma I spoke of earlier is that of working for the love of the kids and not for the love of money. I most certainly do not work for the money and folks think that because you own your own practice you should be rolling in it. Oh, my side, from laughing at this logic.

I have never and will never roll in money and I don't care but I wish I had enough to build a therapy pool at my clinic. I have it all designed and it would be so awesome but alas, my money tree was cut down or something because I can't find it . . . I actually think lightning struck it and it burned down. I'm just thankful for my generous parents who allow me access to their pool over the warm months and that's good enough for me for now.

Again, you can't expect your therapist to be able to provide every cotton-picking medium of treatment out there but this one would be awesome. You may be able to find an aquatic therapy facility in your area though so do take a look and see what's out there.

****

The Dragonfly Approach is my 27 years of experience, trial and error, lack of knowledge early on, passion for learning, a brain that won't quit until it knows, and later on, a husband that told me to go for it. It has taken me this long to feel I finally have a good handle on this OT stuff as well as these OT kids plus, God has been shoving me around a lot lately.

Every therapist will have their approach or method, they will blend different things together and try things maybe I haven't even mentioned yet into their therapy with your kids but not everything works with every therapist's ideas about therapy nor the kid's benefit for that matter.

I do not know everything. I will say, however, that over the years I have learned and studied a great deal and I have been seeing the results and I cannot express how happy it makes me to see one of my OT kids do awesome sauce things, sometimes things completely unexpected.

My approach is from my experience and my heart. It is from a belief that we have to get to the core of the issue and stop throwing pills at everything, stop pretending it's not there because it can get worse, ask the questions I have proposed to you throughout this book, the checklists in the Appendix, and get outside. I have the additional approach of being able to use horses, water, and yoga, but I have a few others that I am excited to introduce to you. They are biofeedback and essential oils.

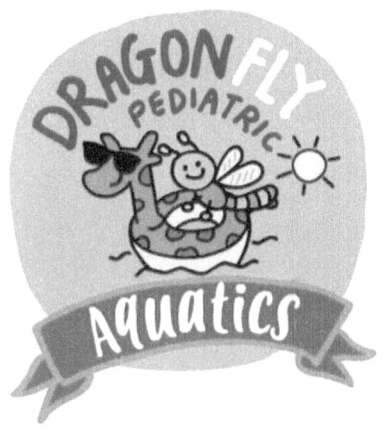

Biofeedback

I am not certified in biofeedback, I will say that from the start but I am versed from tons and tons of reading and studying, experience with it in the clinic, and I use it myself, and on the Professor/husband. I do not have a big fancy machine and I don't offer biofeedback therapy to the general public. What I do though, is use it to introduce a calm to some of my OT kids that have no idea what 'calm' feels like. Not kidding! The biofeedback units I use introduces them to something a lot of them have NEVER felt before. That is nuts. I especially see this in my high on the scale ADHD kids.

First, let's define what biofeedback is: a treatment to basically train the brain using feedback from a device that monitors your breathing and your heart rate. It has been used since the 1960s, kind of fell to the wayside for a bit, but has risen up again, and I love using it with the kids.

Biofeedback has long been used to treat issues such as high blood pressure, muscle tension, and anxiety but I find it very helpful for kids with retained reflexes, ADHD, self-regulation issues, and sensory integration trouble. Pretty much any kid can use biofeedback and I have to say this, that kid that had never felt calm before, demonstrated almost an instant increase in confidence and a self-awareness about his heart and breathing in one session and his mom says he is a different kid since starting biofeedback. Can you imagine not knowing what 'calm' felt like? I couldn't either but then I realized that years ago, when I was a kid, I NEVER felt calm, and that makes me sad for these kids because I remember what it felt like and it's not fun at all!

One of the units that I use, is called 'Inner Balance' by Heartmath. There is an app that can be downloaded for IOS and Android and the unit comes with the appropriate plug for either phone or iPad or other Android devices. The unit clips to your ear lobe and the other end plugs into the phone/iPad/etc. The app runs the person through a series of breathing, centering, and calming. It lets you see your heart rate and then lets you know if you are in the green, calm non-erratic heart rate, or blue, an un-calm erratic heart rate. There are some in-between colors but you get the gist. It lets you know what to do to get your calm and it works great with the OT kids because it is simple. You can find this particular unit at www.heartmath.com.

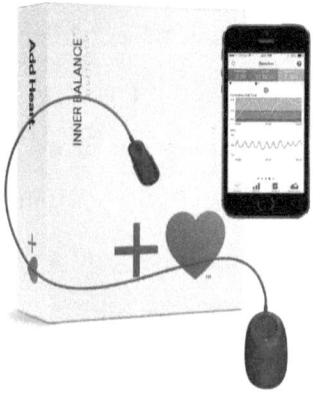

There is another biofeedback unit that I purchased through Amazon Prime and is called 'Muse: The Brain Sensing Headband.' This unit is very intriguing. First, it got a review of 4 stars out of 5 by 516 people who seem very pleased with the unit. Two, it's also a good form of meditation, which is incredibly good for people and children. If you want the direct website for more information it is www.choosemuse.com. The other good thing I see with the Muse is what the company describes about their product: "When you're calm, you'll hear peaceful weather sounds but when your mind wanders, the weather will intensify, guiding you back to a calm state."

The headband literally measures whether your mind is calm or active and translates the data into weather sounds. That is so cool! The Professor has been using it and one thing I have to mention is the more centered you are, the more birds you will hear sing and my awesome husband has heard up to 26 birds sing in one session. I myself have heard none. I've got to get a better handle on my centering as my husband is way better than I am and I'm proud to brag about him!

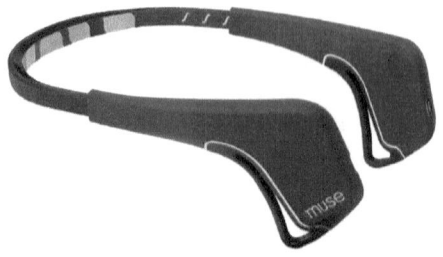

Meditative centering is not done enough by people and children, sometimes I don't do it enough either, though I really try. I know it seems hooey but it's not and there are a ton of great apps for meditation or centering out there. One of my favorites is 'Head Space.' Check it out because it's good.

If you have noticed in the news and such, there is a lot of buzz about the importance of centering, meditation, and relaxation. There are so many things on our planet that take us away from ourselves and thus we lose sight of our importance, lose sight of the fact that our spiritual or soul wellness is important, and our mind's calm is VERY important. You are important and don't forget that. Don't let all the junk in life rob you of the acknowledgment that you are an important part of the big picture of life. The key is to take care of yourself so you can have the best quality of life you can. Do good stuff for you!

Essential Oils

I have to be very frank talking about essential oils. For years I thought they were a form of a New Orleans voodoo witch lady's plot to make more money. I thought, "Who in the heck would get into this stuff and how sad that there are so many people that swear by this. If anyone brings out that purple cool-aide at one of these ridiculous essential oils parties I keep getting invited to, I'm calling the cops."

For years and years, this was my thinking and then God sent me about a dozen people along my life to change my mind and eventually, after getting shoved, kicked, and poked with sticks, I caved and decided to learn all there was to know about this essential oil malarkey and what I found out shamed me yet again.

I have been shamed and humbled more times than our past Presidents have lied. Need I say that this equates to a ton!

Not to mention, I came across that book I spoke of titled 'The Drug Story' and it ticked me off that 'natural' medicine was pushed to the wayside so the 'drugs' could take over. This was done for the love of money. Greed is so ugly!

God does this to me on purpose because He has had a plan for me from the time I was 8 years old. I don't have room here for that story here but let's just say, He has been throwing me curve balls ever since, and although some of them hit me in the face and the heart, they have been worth it, very worth it.

After studying everything I could about these essential oils business and later becoming a certified Aromatherapist, I came across a company that stood out against all of the other overpriced oils as well as the pyramid schemes that are, in my opinion, tainting the essential oils.

My favorite company is called Plant Therapy. They are a small, but growing company out of Idaho that decided against jacking the price up so folks could actually afford it, there's no pyramid scheme, they use 100% pure ingredients, have some awesome products, and allowed me to be a wholesaler for them, though I'm not wholesaling at the moment because my practices have gotten so busy. Remember a few pages back maybe; I mentioned the importance of getting outside into the sun and fresh air? Well, nature was given to us for a reason and that reason is to heal. Think about how you feel when you go to the beach. I know how happy I am when I finally get down there because the drive down stinks and all of a sudden it is as if the population of beachgoers has quadrupled in the last year in my area as we all make our way down. I am haggard, stabby, and stressed by the time we have fought our way down.

Now, I'm this way even before we start the drive because life has a way of beating you down a bit. Not to say I don't love my life, I do, quite a lot, but even my awesome job working with these OT kids and families wears me out a little bit as does my own family and all of their unending needs. I'm ALWAYS thinking and trying to solve various issues with each OT kid so I am giving them my best as well as the best most appropriate therapy plus, I have to solve the woes of my own family, who I love to bits. I have 6 other people to look after in my blended family as well as my two K9 Americans. I also have to grocery shop, clean, exercise, meditate, feed the dogs, find a time to pee, ride the horses, write, blog on my 2 sites, which are called The Blog Blender (theblogblender.com) and the other one is on my website called 'The Dragonfly Blog' (www.dragonflypediatricot.com), etc. You know what I'm talking about; life just wears you thin sometimes.

Back to the beach . . .

After we arrive, and we finally get everything settled into the condo, we've bought the darn groceries (I hate this part because everyone else is buying groceries too in a mad dash to get it over with and do the very thing we all drove down here for in the first place and during the shopping trip, beachgoers can get a little nutty plus, my sensory integration issues are screaming at me at this point), gotten our suits and towels, and as we

FINALLY sink our hinnies into our beach chair . . . aaaaahhhhhh.

The healing of my soul begins as I listen to the sound of the waves hugging the beach, sometimes slapping if they get all riled up from a storm or something, feeling the sand between my toes, watching kids frolic in the water without a care in the world, getting my shumaling on (I'll put that recipe in the Appendix), and just breathing the salty air. Where am I? Out in <u>nature</u>.

Nature was given to us to enjoy, relax in, and as I said, heal! Nature is the beach, the woods, and the plants and flowers, which have been used by Egyptians for over 6,000 years ago for healing.

In a nutshell, aromatherapy (as it is often called) is the practice of using natural essential oils for their many benefits including physical and psychological. However, aromatherapy is even more than just that. The word 'aroma' is a Greek word for spice and this form of 'spice' therapy, if you will, draws upon the awesome healing powers of plants. For thousands of years, before there was modern and harmful medicine, people looked to essential oils for healing and well-being. Our bodies are natural and through these natural essential oils practiced in the form of aromatherapy, we can benefit greatly from the many things that they have to offer.

Have you ever smelled a smell that brought back a flood of memories? For example, when I was about 16 years old, my family and I took a trip to Destin, Florida for our annual beach vacation. All three of us (my 2 sisters and me) were teenagers at the time so teenage boys tended to prowl around us, it was gross, but that's what happened. There were these two brothers this particular year that were quite handsome but good God almighty above they wore so much Polo cologne you could smell them coming 700 miles away. As they neared you, you were overcome with the smell of the smothering Polo and I would gag, my eyes would water, and I felt like I'd fall right out. It was awful. To this day, when I smell a whiff of Polo, I get a bit ill and remember those two boys that we still fondly call "The Polo Brothers."

That's what I mean by a smell bringing back memories. This happens because of our olfactory system (smelling system) and our limbic system (the emotion and drive system). The limbic system, when tickled by a smell, can come to life with past memories because it is the 'emotional' part of our brains.

I get asked all the time what an essential oil is exactly so this is what I say, "These are concentrated aromatic liquids that are obtained from the fruits, seeds, bark, stems, flowers, leaves, or other parts of the plant and you know what else? It is estimated that there are over 10,000 aromatic plants that contain essential oils." I had no idea this number was so high. Did you?

The quality of essential oils is key so be careful what company you go for in this arena. There is actually no organization that oversees the quality of essential oils so if you see the term 'therapeutic grade' on a bottle, it's simply a marketing term so do your homework!

Plant Therapy is a great company and below you will see an impressive timeline of what they have been up to. I love that they make 100% pure essential oils, don't dabble in the pyramid scheme hullabaloo, and don't jack the price up so regular folk, like my OT kids/families and me, can afford them. They also give back to the community and I really dig that. Check out their website at www.planttherapy.com and take a look at their blog, it gives really good information as well.

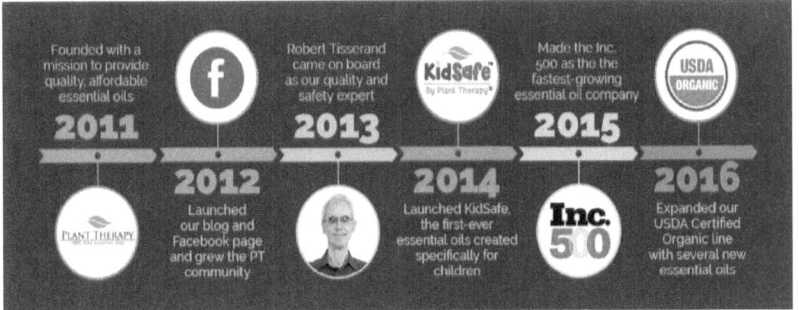

My OT kids and families love Plant Therapy and the roll-on's that are the most popular are A+ Attention, Nighty Night, Tame The Pain, and Calming The Child. All the roll-ons have the directions for application but I tell the parents to roll some on the wrists and have the child rub their wrists together to get it rubbed in good, put some on the back of the neck and rub it in, and if possible, the bottoms of the feet and rub it in.

The A+ Attention is helping my OT kids get through homework easier. Nightly Night is helping calm them to sleep and stay asleep. Tame the Pain has been helping the kids with growing pains. Finally, Calming the Child is being used before a big test at school or any other situation that gives the child anxiety. I am only naming a few but when you check out their website, you will see they have a lot to choose from.

All of the products are awesome at Plant Therapy but I'm giving you the ones I see used in my practice the most, plus I use them in the clinic all the time. I often diffuse the Bouquet essential oil from Plant Therapy in the clinic during OT and EVERYONE loves this. The days I diffuse this, which is often, I notice a lovely calm in each of the kids and their parents. It's really nice to see that relaxation. I also have a Himalayan Salt Lamp, which cleans and purifies the air in my clinic and all of my parents tell me that the air is different in the clinic, cleaner and fresher.

Another thing that impressed me straight off about Plant Therapy is the KidSafe line of products, the roll-on's I mentioned above are from this line and yes, they are truly kid safe. Again, check out their website for a wealth of information and some incredibly great products from an incredibly great and humble company. You'll be glad you did.

Also, check me out on Pinterest as I have loads of additional information about essential oils, as well as tons of other helpful information. It would be under Dragonfly Pediatric Therapy.

The Team

This is a bit of an updated chapter, as I have taken on a third clinic a little over a year ago. In addition to my home clinic, I work at a school-based clinic and now I'm at a Neurodevelopment clinic with several wonderful professionals who I call, 'The Team.' I just love it there and have learned so much from them.

The reason I took on this additional clinic is that we have such a great need in our town, as I have mentioned before. The director of this clinic asked me to be their OT and I saw a wonderful opportunity to work around other professionals as I have been solo for over 21 years. Working at this clinic has been eye-opening and has taught me a lot about the importance of 'The Team.'

So, you may ask, "Why would my child with special needs need a whole team?" Well, because of the complexity of each case, a set of professionals can sure help make things a lot easier and more understandable. Let me tell you what usually happens first, though.

First, you may start to notice that something is off. Your child doesn't seem to be developing like your other child did or you notice that your only child doesn't seem to be where his/her peers are. Another scenario, one that I see a lot, is that your child was developing just fine with good eye contact, speech, and they were eating well and then all of a sudden, things started going backward. In other words, your incredible parental instincts kick in and you KNOW something isn't right.

For some of you, you will go to your pediatrician and point it out to them. Some of the docs are more versed than others and will immediately suggest that you have them 'tested' to see what is going on or seek an OT or ST (speech therapy), every situation is different. Other docs and I hear this way too much, will tell you everything is okay and that you are just worried over nothing. This last one ticks me off because you feel discounted and that's not a good feeling at all. I liken it to

221

when my brand-new car was making a weird noise, I take it in, which is a pain because I need my car and not having it for 3 days was not fun, and long story short, they tell me that everything is fine and they don't hear the noise. This infuriates me because it makes me feel as if they think I'm making it up and bringing my car in is loads of fun! Not to say your child is a car but you get my point. No one likes to be discounted ESPECIALLY if you are talking about your human child that you love beyond reason.

A neuropsychological evaluation may be recommended if your child displays difficulties or abrupt changes in memory, thinking, personality, speech, or other behaviors which interfere with their daily living and/or development. Part of this evaluation is done by what is called a psychometrist. A psychometrist is highly trained in administrating and scoring various tests that assess your child's neuropsychological functioning. Psychometrists work under the supervision of a licensed clinical psychologist.

At our clinic, a child will come in for most of the day and the psychometrist will administer several tests to try and determine what might be going on. Once the testing is done, the tests are scored, and then the findings are interpreted by our clinical psychologist who will provide a diagnosis, if there is one, and write up a very detailed report with recommendations. The family will meet with her to go over the findings and come up with a plan to best help this child and his/her family on this new journey they may find themselves on.

In many cases, OT is recommended, especially if it is a diagnosis of autism, ADHD, ADD, sensory processing, dyslexia, and many more that I see each day. If there is a delay in speech then speech therapy will be recommended as well. Our speech therapist is awesome and I love it when we have a child together because we can collaborate and give each other a lot of information to help this child out in the best way possible. We also may co-treat, which is when we treat a child together, which can benefit certain children who may not be able to tolerate 2 separate therapies or we feel they would benefit better with both of us there.

In some cases, physical therapy may be recommended, though we don't have a PT at our clinic because we don't usually see a child with this type of therapy need. Pediatric physical therapists help children who may have problems moving and performing other physical activities. They help treat issues like injuries, pre-existing conditions, and other problems caused by illness or disease.

Some kids have a combination of issues and therefore may need additional therapies other than the ones I just mentioned.

Applied Behavior Analysis (ABA) is recommended for those children who are having behavior issues. ABA therapy is based on the science of learning and behavior. The ultimate goal is to increase the behaviors that are helpful and decrease the behaviors that are harmful or affecting functioning and learning in society and school. We have an ABA therapist at our clinic and she is wonderful. She provides things such as ABA consultation and parent training. She also connects children with the best ABA services for their needs and abilities and is an Individualized Educational Plan or IEP advocate. An IEP is a map that lays out the program of special education instruction and is designed to meet a child's exact needs. Parents often find that navigating this can be daunting so an IEP advocate can really be helpful.

Sometimes, a child is having a lot of emotional trouble that may go along with their diagnosis and in this case, counseling may be recommended. When I was struggling with my own issues (ADHD, dyslexia, retained reflexes, and SPD) I wish I could have had counseling because when I hit that wall of depression in high school, it was really bad. I'm sure if I had asked my mom, she would have taken me, but it just didn't dawn on me at the time.

We have a couple of counselors at our clinic as well. One of them specializes in small children specifically and has this interesting certification called Parent-Child Interaction Therapy or PCIT. PCIT is a combination of play therapy (which I will mention more in a bit) and behavioral therapy for young children and their parents/caregivers. The parent/caregivers learn and practice techniques for relating to their child who may be dealing with emotional or behavior problems, language issues, developmental disabilities, or mental health disorders. PCIT is used a lot with kids on the autism spectrum but can also be used with kids who have experienced trauma.

Play therapy is another therapy that your child may need as a part of their team. The Association for Play Therapy defines play therapy as "the systematic use of a theoretical model to establish an interpersonal process wherein trained play therapists use the therapeutic powers of play to help clients prevent or resolve psychosocial difficulties and achieve optimal growth and development." Play is the language of a child. It's fun and elevates the child's spirit and mood. It helps with their self-expression and self-knowledge.

Hence, play is a perfect medium to use in a therapeutic way to help with any psychosocial issues they may be having. We don't have a play therapist at the clinic but have a few that we refer to when it becomes necessary. I'm currently studying Child-Centered Play Therapy as part of my continuing education and it's quite fascinating. I do a lot of play therapy in OT and didn't realize it until I started my current studies.

So, here are the members of the team you might find your child a part of:

-Pediatrician

-Psychometrist

-Clinical Psychologist

-Occupational Therapist

-Speech Therapist

-Physical Therapist (not so much in my clinic)

-ABA Therapist

-Counselor

-Play Therapist

I'd also like to mention the use of Music Therapy. Music just makes everyone feel good and I know in OT I use it quite often but there are trained Music Therapists out there who are very good at what they do. Music therapy is defined by the Canadian Association for Music Therapy as "the skillful use of music and musical elements by an accredited music therapist to promote, maintain, and restore mental, physical, emotional, and spiritual health. Music has nonverbal, creative, structural, and emotional qualities. These are used in the therapeutic relationship to facilitate contact, interaction, self-awareness, learning, self-expression, communication, and personal development."

Your child's team can consist of all of the above or a select few. My goal was to give you some information about what you may hear mentioned or come across on your own. Remember, if a member of your team is not sitting well with you, move on because your team is yours and is an important part of your child's life.

Things to Avoid in Your Child's Diet

Now, I am not a registered dietician but I am a certified Nutritional Therapist, I am a pediatric OT who has 27 years under her belt, I have had and have solved my own gut issues, plus I have kids of my own who have tummy issues at times. I've also dedicated the last 2 years of my life to studying this topic.

First, you have to realize that our intestines make up at least if not more than 70% of our immunity system. That's a big deal!!! That's why gut health is very very important!

Clean eating is when you avoid those foods that the food people load up with junk that is not only not good for us like GMO's, MSG, and artificial sweeteners, but can make us quite sick. This poison is literally altering our DNA, creating new syndromes and diagnoses, and making us all fat.

If I had my way, I'd grow all of my food and raise my own fish, turkey, and chicken but I'm not a farmer, I am an OT so that isn't possible at this time in my life. If you can, do it because that way you can dictate what is in your food. You wouldn't spray chemical junk on your garden. You'd probably hand-weed or de-bug it yourself or use other natural gardening methods. If you can't garden, then try going to a whole foods market or a farmer's market and buy good clean food for you and your family.

There are several bad things that they do to our food and I'm not going to go into all of them because honestly, I'm not familiar with everything and maybe I don't want to know for fear of fainting.

Years and years ago, when they weren't trying to cheat and make more money by adding hormones, antibiotics, and whatever the heck else they put into our food so they could crank it out faster, there wasn't really a huge man-made internal 'platform' inadvertently laid down for bodily chaos to launch off of.

Fast forward to now . . . there are all kinds of junk in our foods both at the grocery stores and restaurants, though several companies are improving and changing this, waves from all of our electronics, bad air we are breathing, depending on where you live, a huge increase in the number of vaccinations recommended, women aren't breastfeeding long enough or at all because they've got to get back to work (I didn't mention this earlier but breastfeed your children if you can and be sure you are eating clean while doing it, PLEASE, it is so good for them and shoot for at least 6 months if you can't go any longer), and many other things I have mentioned already.

These things set an unsavory internal platform that was not there before. So, let's think about this and I have mentioned this before:

-What was the mother eating before and during pregnancy?

-What has her husband been up to before he met his wife? What is he eating?

-Both parents more than likely had vaccinations, which adds to things.

-How much technology are they being exposed to?

-Was the pregnancy stressful, did she get sick, or did she have a C-section?

-Did she breastfeed?

-When your baby starts to eat table food, are you giving your baby GMO (genetically modified organisms), gluten, MSG, GMO-ridden soy and corn, or cow's milk? Did you eat these before and during pregnancy? Probably, but you didn't know any better, until now!

So, you see a <u>layered complex internal platform</u> has been laid down because of all of this. No, don't do it, don't blame yourself, we are just now getting a handle on this information.

The Professor and I like to watch the show 'Naked and Afraid' sometimes. These crazy people amaze me exposing themselves and their body parts, if

233

you know what I mean, to the elements. If you haven't seen an episode, watch one so you get what I'm about to say.

Picture this, on the drive into the start of the show, the man and woman (in separate trucks) are each talking to the camera dude about how excited and/or nervous they are and why they think they can be a good partner and make it to day 21. They also discuss their take on nudity and what their family members must think. They are happy, they are hopeful, and they are rearing to go.

Once they each arrive at the designated drop off spot, they strip, throw their clothes into the back of the truck they came in on, and make their way into the forest, woods, beach, etc. to meet up with their new partner who they will try to survive with for 21 days. They will also each get a sack that has a few items in it like the map of the area and a tool that they chose and felt would help the both of them over the next 21 days. Most bring a fire starter, a huge machete, or a pot to boil water in. A dude brought duct tape one time and I thought that was genius.

Okay, so they come in hydrated, fed, clothed, warm, happy, determined, nervous, and excited.

The first 'layer' is being added as they tromp through their environment looking for a good place for their 'camp.' They slowly become dehydrated as they are breathing or in some cases panting, depending on their level of physical readiness because as you breathe, water is expelled. They are sweating too, adding to their dehydration. They are also getting bit by a ton of bugs, which irritates them to death, again, they are butt naked so any part of their exposed epidermis is a feast for the bugs. They may step on a thorn or a swarm of ants that stab or bite the stew out of them . . . another layer. They finally find a spot and it's gotten dark so they are only focused on their shelter at this point, which they manage to get pieced together and then they 'try' and fall asleep. The bugs are so bad as well as the noise of the environment, that they both sleep terribly, and another layer is added.

They wake up, if they have slept at all, crabby, hungry, thirsty, and slightly stabby. They work all morning on making a fire to help ward off some of the bugs so they can maybe sleep and boil water to drink if they can even find some. Some partners manage a fire and some don't. Some find water and some don't. Some find food and some don't. This all builds layers onto this 'platform.'

So, through this layer-by-layer process that is being laid down because of the circumstances they have put themselves in, it can either build a platform of success or failure.

Soon, they are so dehydrated, they start fighting with each other, they are crying, they run off to be by themselves, they are hungry, they aren't sleeping, they are cold, they feel sick, etc.

All of a sudden, a monsoon comes onto their island, for example, and they are trapped in their pitiful shelter for days and days, yet another layer of isolation, hunger, being cold, etc.

And then . . . one of them gets incredibly ill from whatever and they start throwing up uncontrollably or having chronic diarrhea. All of those layers that have set-up this platform for either success or failure, pushes one of them to the dreaded failure point and they make the choice of tapping out thus not making the whole 21 days with their partner.

The other player pushes on even though he/she had that same platform up to this point, but that last thing that defeated their partner didn't befall them. They succeed.

Now, you might have already figured out what I'm getting at. If so, you are one smart cookie.

This is the same platform that is created by all of the things I have already listed. All of the things I have mentioned for a kid might shakedown and maybe one item sets the whole thing in motion such as vaccines, as some wholeheartedly believe. However, it could be a number of factors that we are just now uncovering so I can't solely blame vaccinations.

However, I will say this, vaccines have been known to cause the following:

1. Encephalitis

2. Seizures

3. Immune system deficiencies

4. Gastrointestinal issues

5. ADHD*

6. Autism*

*More specific information on these last two can be found in the book called 'Medical Medium' by Anthony William.

-Now, encephalitis is horrible and can cause severe pain, mood swings, inattention, aggression, impulsivity, and balance issues.

-Seizures can cause alterations in conciseness, mood swings, and impulsivity.

-Immune system deficiencies can cause children to have more bacterial infections such as UTIs and ear infections. It can also cause them to have more viral infections such as fevers of unknown origin and gastrointestinal disturbances.

-Gastrointestinal damage can cause diarrhea, reflux, vomiting, and gastroesophageal reflux disease (GERD). It can also cause more susceptibility to viral and bacterial diseases, which then requires antibiotics, and antibiotics in your system can kill the healthy flora in your gut.

So, yes, vaccinations for one kid may have set that 'platform' off in the form of autism, for example, but for another, diet could have been a culprit, and maybe what's causing him/her to look as if they have ADHD. My point is, we are just now starting to understand certain things. As I said, an internal platform is set and when that last 'ingredient' is introduced in certain kids, then things seem to go amiss. It just depends on the layering of the initial 'platform.' Does that make sense?

There are several things in our foods (and a couple of foods I mention specifically below because they are in practically everything) that are not helping these kids or even our adult selves for that matter:

-GMO'S (genetically modified organisms-need I say more?)

-GLUTEN (a protein found in certain grains like wheat, barley, rye, and spelt; it can cause inflammation, especially in the intestinal tract and bowel)

-DAIRY (certain dairy is very high in fat which can hurt your liver; lactose in dairy combined with fat and sugar negatively affects overall health; dairy also causes an increase in mucus and is a major cause of inflammation and allergies; I tell all of my OT families to switch to almond and/or coconut milk)

-MSG'S (monosodium glutamate, which is a food additive; can cause inflammation, swelling, kills brain cells, can make you feel confused and anxious, plus a whole lot more)

-SOY (GMO's have destroyed soy and almost any soy product can contain MSG; can cause breast cancer, internal body inflammation, low sperm count in men; for little kids, you may see boobs on very young girls and boys too)

-CORN (GMO's have also destroyed corn; can cause increased inflammation; feeds viruses, mold, fungus, and bacteria that may be lurking inside your body)

-ARTIFICIAL SWEETENERS (act as neurotoxins because they contain aspartame which can disrupt neurons and your central nervous system)

-DYES (can cause cancer, hyperactivity, allergies, hypersensitivity, and asthma just to name a few)

I would avoid these at all costs not just for your kids but also for EVERYONE! If something is genetically modified and God didn't have a hand in it, steer clear!

'Gluten,' for example, is derived from the glue-like property it has that gives dough, for example, its elastic property. Some people's bodies think this is an invader, and long story short, because it thinks it's an invader, the series of events the body does causes a degeneration of the intestinal wall.

Moreover, did you know that we are the only species that continues to drink ANOTHER ANIMAL'S milk long after it is necessary? Sit and think that through for a minute. No other mammal continues to drink its mother's milk let alone an entirely different animal's milk. You know why? Because our bodies were not designed to digest another animal's milk, why would it? Cow's milk is also a protein that the body thinks is an invader and then there's more intestinal damage.

Most kids with special needs have a very sensitive digestive system anyway so really consider eating clean and avoiding the things that I just threw out there. Your gut will thank you plus you will see good things happen to your kids like boosting immunity, improving neurological functioning, healing the bowel, killing candida, better sleep, reducing anxiety and depression, and possibly improving autism and ADHD! I'm here to tell you folks that I have seen these last two firsthand from several kids on my caseload. It's amazing!

One thing to know, in addition to the things I mentioned before about things that cause an unhealthy gut, other things may come into play too: chronic stress, toxins, and an imbalance between beneficial and harmful bacteria in your gut, that's why probiotics are pushed a lot these days but do some good research here or consult a dietician just for good measure for the right one (I like and recommend Mary Ruth's Liquid Probiotic-on Amazon). Also, your brain's function and your gut are connected and if your gut is not healthy, it WILL affect the way your brain functions.

Did you know that there are GMOs in certain baby formulas and baby foods? I didn't either and that is alarming and really ticks me off!

Jane Goodall, that awesome primate-loving lady who went on a quest to save them once said, "How could we have ever believed that it was a good idea to grow our food with poisons?" No sh*t, Jane, I concur!!

I suggest a meeting with a pediatric dietician who specializes in kids with special needs and make a diet plan that will work for your kid. What we put in our bodies is of utmost importance, I promise you that. The saying, "You are what you eat," should really be, "You will have a better overall body and a better output if you

put into it only the things that are pure and good for it."
Wouldn't you agree?

****

Have you ever heard of 'oxidative stress?' What this means is an imbalance between the production of free radicals and the ability of the body to detoxify their harmful effects through neutralization by antioxidants. Um, what?

Have you ever had brain fog, sluggishness, depression, upset tummy, etc.? Those are just a few signs of oxidative stress and that you are eating the wrong things. Bruce Ames, Ph.D. of the National Institute of Environmental Health Sciences Center says, "In each human cell, DNA is hit about 10,000 times per day by mutagenic oxidants." To this I say, why are we seeing so many genetic disorders all of a sudden . . . this is why!

I'm not trying to freak you out but I want you to be aware that again, you are what you eat and if you are eating junk, your body will produce junk and make you very sick. Don't starve your brain and body of health, which was so intricately strung together by God, because it's the only one you get. I know it's not always easy especially with all the stuff we pile on ourselves to make a life and a living but if your quality of life that you are working so hard for isn't measuring up, you might want to rethink a few things.

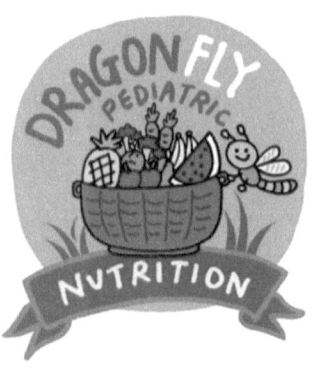

I have to touch on something that I don't have all of the answers to because I don't specialize in feeding issues. Back in my day, Speech Therapists addressed this but I know that more and more OTs are now a part of this. So, if your child has feeding issues which means they won't eat anything other than a select few foods, usually carbohydrates, and you are worried about their nutrition, please seek out a therapist that specializes in this.

I do have some information I can give here specific to autism and ADHD. As of now, there is a movement to cut out grains and sugars in these kid's diets, this is great but only if fruit is taking the place of the sugars that are being omitted. The other trend is the ketogenic diet. Any improvement that you see in your child will only be temporary while following this diet and in the end can cause adrenal fatigue.

For those kids who are drawn to high-sugar foods and high-calorie starches, such as French fries and chicken nuggets, there is a misinterpretation of what the body is asking for. Kids with ADHD and autism use extremely large amounts of glucose, which is the brain's primary food. The misinterpretation is that the glucose can be obtained from high-sugar foods and high-calorie starches which is NOT what the child needs. Instead, they should be eating as much fruit as possible. Fruit has the molecularly structured glucose that their brain needs, NOT the junk which probably has GMO's, MSG's, and some of the other things I have named, which in turn, makes everything worse. So, if you have a carb crazy kid, push fruit as much as possible instead of the junk. The fruits I recommend are bananas, red apples, red grapes, melon, mango, papaya, coconut, pears, and berries.

I also recommend picking up Anthony William's book titled, 'Life-Changing Foods.'

My Own Life-Changing Diet Journey

Something horrible happened to me a few years ago that changed my life forever and changed the way that I now treat my OT kids. Though it was quite debilitating and painful, pain that lasted over a year, it has been well worth it. I include this chapter in this book because I want to knock home how a change in your diet can have profound effects on you and your child's quality of life and overall health.

Here's the story . . .

So, the Professor and I had noticed that our backs were getting sorer and sorer each time we woke up from a pitiful night's sleep and enough was enough, as I was functioning poorly because of it. In discussing this with him, I discovered that the mattress that I inherited when we got married, was something like 20 years old. I barfed in my mouth a little bit when I heard this. I had a little extra money, so I offered to buy a new one because

249

I was no longer going to sleep on this 20-year-old mattress that probably had so much human skin in it, we could have resurrected another human being or two. He agreed so we ordered a brand-new mattress and eagerly awaited its arrival.

Our mattress came a few days after ordering it and laid on the driveway for several hours before one of my strong kids came home from school to help us lug it into the house. It was one of those memory foam ones that came rolled up into itself and wrapped in plastic. We wrestled the fossilized one out and happily chucked it onto the curb and eagerly replace it with our new one with the expectation of the greatest sleep of our lives because that's what the ratings on it said. Later that night, with fresh sheets on our new mattress/bed and high expectations, we went to sleep.

The next morning, I turned to my husband, who had just entered the bathroom as I exited the shower, and said, "Holy cow, honey! I slept like a dream! What about you?" As I looked at him, waiting for his take on his night of sleep on the new mattress, I noticed a strange look on his face. He grabbed his glasses and turned my fresh from the shower body around so my back was facing the mirror and said, "What the heck bit you?" As I craned my neck to see what he was talking about, I was startled to see one large ugly welt that was kind of purple, pink, and gray all at once just to the left of my spine over my kidney area. We deduced that I must have been bitten by one mean spider, not realizing at the time that yes, it was a spider, and a poisonous one at that and it was in our bed. The next night, I was bitten two more times on the back of my right hand. Funny thing, the Professor wasn't bitten at all, just me, but for very good reason.

When all was said and done, we discovered that I had been bitten by a Brown Recluse spider a total of three times and what transpired after these bites was, to put it mildly, horrendous and would completely change the way I was doing things, as I tried to find answers on how to heal naturally. (Oh, and by the way, we found the little cuss that bit me and made sure he never returned again.)

Now, the spider bite not only triggered the Lyme's Disease virus I apparently had, which was lying dormant up until that moment, it also kicked up the Epstein Barr virus that I had inherited from my mom, who got it from her mom. My grandma had severe rheumatoid arthritis and EBV can be the underlying cause of this. She may have had Lyme's disease too, but we have no record of that.

Around the time I was bit, I was seeing a really cool OT kid whose mom was very progressive when it came to natural healing and had been suffering from various ailments herself like joint pain, horrible gut issues, and whispers of possible autoimmune issues. She was not at all interested in this Western Medical model so, by the grace of God, she came across a series of books written by Anthony William aka The Medical Medium, and highly recommended I take a look at them in order to heal. God sent her my way right when I needed her, I can tell you that.

If any of you are familiar with this guy, you will know that he has a very special relationship with The Spirit of the Most High, who he fondly calls, Spirit. Without getting to nuts into detail about this guy, as it is best to read his books, I will give you a brief run-down of why he and his Spirit pal, saved my life after the spider bite, as I was deathly ill, I can assure you. I will also tell you how I incorporated his information into my practice with my OT kids and how I now aggressively address diet with every one of them. I fondly call the pairing of these two, 'Spanthony'-Spirit and Anthony mashed together.

Now, before I go on, there are A LOT of naysayers out there with regard to Spanthony's recommendations and I too doubted when my OT kid's mom introduced me to his books, but as I began to read and apply some of the things that I was learning from his first book titled, 'Medical Medium: Secrets Behind

Chronic and Mystery Illness and How to Finally Heal,' I not only began healing from the aftermath of the Brown Recluse bites, but a lot of what he was talking about made a lot of sense to my way of thinking and my entire life changed exponentially. I am living proof of what Spanthony has been trying to share with the world. Living proof!

Here's what I mean . . .

Not only was I extremely sick and in severe pain from the spider bites plus, I was living with super ticked off Epstein Barr and Lyme's disease viruses (yes, Lyme's disease is a virus, not a bacteria), I also had high blood pressure (on meds for it), depression (on meds for it), ADHD (on meds for it), and had gotten chubby again because my liver was very sick as well. Though I didn't know that last one until a bit later on. Plus, my gut was a mess and at the time, I thought I had leaky gut which was causing irritable bowel syndrome, severe abdominal pain, and constant diarrhea, though this became much worse after the spider bite. My quality of life was not good and I was at one of the lowest points in my life, though I didn't let a lot of people know this. I was also missing a lot of work, something that I DO NOT like to do as the OT kids count on me being there for them.

I will tell you what the symptoms are of Epstein-Barr and Lyme's disease viruses and I will also explain to you how it affected my life. However, I am only touching on a small portion of what Spanthony has in his books so I do urge you to continue your studies using the books he has out there on Amazon.

First, Epstein-Barr virus (EBV). There are over 60 varieties of this virus and they present themselves in four different stages, I won't go into them here because he explains it best. You can get it from your mom if she has it, from infected blood, eating out (if the cook has it, cuts his/her finger, and accidentally bleeds into your food), through bodily fluids, and through kissing believe it or not. If you have it, it can worsen with certain life situations like puberty, pregnancy, or menopause. For me, although I didn't know it at the time, my EBV got really bad while I was pregnant with my daughter. I hurt all over and towards the end, I thought I had a combination of carpal tunnel syndrome and tennis elbow in both arms/hands so I slept very little for the last two months of my pregnancy due to the burning, tingling, and numbness. This is not what was going on but that's what I thought was going on because it was what I was told by my doc. It was awful!

Epstein-Barr virus symptoms can be misdiagnosed but the underlying cause is actually this virus so bear with me:

-Lupus

-Hypothyroidism and other thyroid diseases

-Chronic Fatigue syndrome

-Fibromyalgia

-Tinnitus

-Vertigo and Meniere's disease

-Anxiety

-Dizziness

-Chest tightness

-Esophageal spasms

-Asthma

-Insomnia

-Tingling and numbness of the hands and feet

-Heart palpitations

After the spider bite, these were the symptoms I was dealing with: severe anxiety, pain all over, numbness, burning, and tingling of the arms and hands so bad that I didn't have any grip strength, a lot of dizziness so bad that I would feel severe motion sickness, esophageal spasms, fibromyalgia type symptoms, chronic fatigue (which really stunk because I experienced this on our 'whole' family trip to Wyoming right after the bite and it made the vacation very challenging), severe chest tightness that would happen at night and I would feel like my lungs were collapsing, and severe heart palpitations that made me feel like I would pass out. This spider bite triggered and made worse the viruses I already had and made my life a living hell but because I followed all of Spanthony's advice, I fully healed from these viruses in exactly 1 year and three months.

Now, let's talk about Lyme's disease. Again, Lyme's disease is a virus, not a bacteria as many have believed. A bacteria does not cause neurological disturbances but a virus, like Lyme's, can. Lyme's disease can be misdiagnosed, just like EBV, and causes a lot of suffering believe me. First, there are several things that can trigger your once dormant Lyme's disease and they are:

-Mold

-Mercury-based dental fillings

-Mercury in other forms like frequently eating seafood and vaccinations

-Pesticides and herbicides

-Insecticides in your home

-A stressful event like a death in the family

-Spider bites

-Bee stings

-Tick bite (again, insect bites don't give you this

virus but can trigger it)

-Certain prescription medicines

-Recreational drug abuse

Some symptoms of Lyme's disease can be:

-Twitching

-Spasms

-Fatigue

-Brain fog

-Memory loss

-Nerve and joint pain

-Muscle weakness

-Restless leg syndrome

-Swelling

-Tingling in the hands and feet

And just like EBV, your symptoms can be misdiagnosed as:

-Multiple Sclerosis

-Lupus

-Fibromyalgia

-Rheumatoid Arthritis

-Chronic Fatigue syndrome

Now, I know this is a lot to take in and it was for me too but I was so sick, in severe pain all over, literally felt like I was dying, and needed answers. What I knew without a doubt is that I wanted to heal but I wanted to do it naturally because I had some run-ins with synthetic medications in the past. For example, in order to keep my over 40-year-old self from getting pregnant again, I decided to jump on the birth control pill wagon. Long story short, the birth control pill, paired with severe stress finally coming to an end after 16 long years (my failed marriage), caused an 'explosion' in my body which, in turn, caused every hair on my body to fall out. This phenomenon is called telogen effluvium which is severe or total hair loss due to severe stress or can be from synthetic medications, as I, unfortunately, found out. I have blogged about what happened to me, as that is what I do for my own mental therapy, and what I found out was that I was not alone in this hair loss nightmare.

There was a ton of comments from other women out there who had this happen to them and had the same combination that I had. So, I was absolutely NOT going to turn to synthetic drugs again. Plus, I did not like the side effects of my depression and ADHD medications. They seemed to be outweighing the benefits.

So, here is what I did. From the books I have mentioned, I learned what fed these viruses in my body, how to detox my body of heavy metals, I also learned that because I had done the high protein/fat low carb diet for so many years, I had created a fatty and sluggish liver and I had to heal this too in the process in order for all of this to work, I learned what foods, supplements, herbal teas, and tinctures I had to include in my diet every day. I also learned the power of celery juice.

Before I go on, however, I want to briefly touch on why the liver is the most important organ in your body. I will keep it brief because there is A LOT on the liver and Spanthony's book titled 'Liver Rescue' is an excellent source to learn more about your liver. Because of Spanthony, I take more care of my liver than ever before. I also have told my liver that I am sorry for treating it so bad for so many years, yes, I talk to my liver, I'm weird, it's just who I am.

Now, the liver is the most amazing, powerful, and hardest working organ in our bodies. As I have mentioned, I caused my liver to be fatty and sluggish because of the high-fat diet I decided to do years ago plus, I had suffered from eczema for years, which is a result of a ticked-off liver. Having a fatty or sluggish liver or a liver that is beaten down by toxins or too much protein or fat in your diet can be the root of about every symptom and condition known to man including acne, constipation, dark circles under the eyes, fatigue, emotional issues, irritable bowel syndrome, inflammation, pain, liver cancer, eczema, psoriasis, insomnia, seasonal affect disorder, sinus infections, urinary tract infections, and weight gain.

Interestingly, the liver is composed of three depths. You can read more about these depths in

Anthony William's book titled 'Live Rescue.' Each depth has an important job to do to keep our body clean and healthy on the inside. Our livers are designed to deal with some of the junk we throw at it but problems begin to arise when the liver is flooded or bogged down with too many toxins and it can't keep us safe from all of them, even though it is constantly doing the best it can. We have to throw our livers a 'bone' so it can work in the way it was designed for our health.

To start, I had to get rid of all of the junk that I was eating which was feeding the EBV and Lyme's disease and really messing up my gut health. This included: MSG, dairy, canola oil, artificial flavors, gluten, pork, citric acid, soy, corn, processed beat sugar, farmed fish, natural flavors, eggs, and artificial sweeteners. I also added celery juice and a heavy metal detox smoothie each morning for breakfast. Let me talk about celery juice specifically for a moment and please note, Spanthony has a book out titled 'Celery Juice' which is game-changing so please get your hands on this book!

When I first learned about celery juice my first thought was, "Eck, who in the heck drinks this, and what in the world will it do to help me?" Well, it has changed so much about my health, I'd have to write another book on it, so I'll keep it simple. The health benefits of celery juice include:

-Lowers inflammation

-Supports weight-loss

-Aids digestion

-Reduces bloating and small intestine bowel obstruction

-Fights infection

-Helps prevent UTI's

-Helps heal acne

-Prevents high blood pressure

-Helps lower cholesterol

-Helps prevent ulcers

-Protects liver health by neutralizing and flushing out toxins

-Helps gum, teeth, and mouth problems

-Helps chronic acid reflux

-Fights autoimmune disease

-Helps restore adrenal glands

-The sodium clusters in celery juice helps reverse illnesses

-Helps eradicate strep bacteria

-Kills EBV and Shingles

-Brings down toxic liver heat

-Repairs hydrochloric acid and liver bile production

     Celery juice contains these things called mineral salts which are very important for our bodies to perform at their best. These mineral salts are the reason that all of the above happens when you drink 16 ounces (Spanthony says up to 30 ounces) of straight celery juice, with no pulp, on an empty stomach, first thing in the morning, and waiting 15-30 minutes before eating anything else, preferably a non-fat breakfast, please see 'Liver Rescue.' For me and the Professor, I make each of us about 16 ounces of celery juice every morning, we both drink it on an empty stomach, I down mine immediately, and the Professor sips his for a bit. After I clean the juicer and then make our heavy metal detox smoothies, about 20 minutes have passed so the celery juice can do its healing.

An aside, the Professor has cleared up his acid reflux, rid himself of depression, lowered his cholesterol and blood pressure, his tummy trouble is nearly gone (nearly because sometimes he gets ahold of 'junk' food and he stirs it all up again), he's sleeping better than ever, and has more energy than I have ever seen since introducing celery juice to him.

Now, the heavy metal detox smoothie is another key in healing because heavy metals are poison to our bodies. They can cause such things as ADHD, ADD, autism, depression, obsessive-compulsive disorders, mood disorders, Alzheimer's, concentration issues, memory loss, and for me, they were feeding the EBV and Lyme's disease. Heavy metals are food for many viruses in our bodies, not just the aforementioned. The heavy metals I am referring to are lead, mercury, aluminum, arsenic, nickel, cadmium, and copper. They can build up in our bodies by our own exposure and can be passed down to us from generation to generation, especially mercury which can stick around in the bloodline for millennia. You may wonder how one can acquire heavy metals by our own hands, as you really can't help what you inherited from your ancestors.

When was the last time you drank from an aluminum can, used aluminum foil, had a vaccination, lived in a house with old copper pipes, drank water from your tap, or went out for a walk and the city had just treated the area with pesticides? It's everywhere I'm afraid but by drinking the heavy metal detox smoothie, you can help flush these horrible culprits out and put yourself on the road to better health.

I recommend the heavy detox smoothie to nearly all of my OT kids and their families, I say nearly all because some of them already know about it and have been doing it for quite some time. This makes me so happy. Here is the recipe:

-2 banana

-2 cups of Wyman's Wild Blueberries (in the

frozen food section)

-4 dropperfuls of cilantro alcohol-free tincture or 1 cup of fresh cilantro (Spanthony says fresh cilantro but I don't always have this on hand so I use a tincture, I'm not sure what his take is on this but it seems to be working regardless)

-1 cup pure orange juice not from concentrate

-1 teaspoon barley grass juice powder

-1 teaspoon spirulina

-1 small handful of Atlantic dulse flakes

This recipe above makes a lot so you might share it with a friend or family member or you can half it for a single serving or you can save some for later. The trifecta of this recipe, from what I understand, is the barley grass juice, spirulina, and dulse, as these three work together to grab the heavy metals, transport them, and then exit them out of the body. Again, if you read the books I have recommended and that are listed in the References, you will get the whole picture. Also, make sure you are getting the right products by visiting www.medicalmedium.com. Under the blogs tab, there is a search box, type in 'Detox Smoothie,' and he will give you links to the products he recommends.

So, in addition to cutting out certain foods and additives, drinking my celery juice every morning on an empty stomach, and drinking my smoothie every morning, there were certain foods that I made sure I ate nearly every day as well as several herbs and supplements. For now, I'm just going to list the food that

I included in my diet and just a few supplements and herbs I used as they are very specific to what is going on with you and again, you have to read his books to understand. The following is some of what I did to combat my EBV and Lyme's disease:

-Wild blueberries in my detox smoothie everyday

-Celery juice every morning on an empty stomach

-Asparagus

-Spinach

-Cilantro in my detox smoothie every morning

-Coconut oil

-Garlic

-Ginger tea

-Raspberries and raspberry tea

-Papayas

-Cucumbers

-Kale

-Cinnamon in my detox smoothie every morning

-Onions

-Butter lettuce

   Some of the supplements and herbs I used and use:

-Cat's claw alcohol-free tincture

-Zinc

-Vitamin B12

-Licorice root alcohol-free tincture

-Lemon balm alcohol-free tincture and tea

-5-MTHF

-Selenium

-L-lysine

-Spirulina in my detox smoothie every day

-Ester-C

-Nettle leaf

-Thyme

-Reishi mushrooms

-Nascent iodine

My point in listing all of this is to show you that it is all-natural. Part of the naysayer complaints is that Spanthony is telling you to get off of all of your medications and do these whacko things to heal, which is not at all true. It is all-natural otherwise, I would NOT be following it plus, I wouldn't be recommending certain aspects to my OT kids and their families.

In discovering that my liver was fatty and sluggish, there was a whole bunch of things that I learned and did from the book 'Liver Rescue.' The first thing I learned was to lower my fat intake substantially, especially first thing in the morning so my liver could do the other things it needed to do and not have to contend with a whole bunch of fat.

So, some of the foods that I also included was:

-Apples

-Bananas

-Broccoli

-Berries

-Brussel sprouts

-Coconut (but not in the morning as it has some fats)

-Cranberries

-Dandelion Greens in the form of herbal tea

-Dates

-Figs

-Purple grapes

-Lemons and limes

-Mangoes

-Melons

-Mushrooms

-Oranges and tangerines

-Raw honey (which I use to sweeten my detox smoothie)

-100% organic maple syrup (which I use to sweeten my detox smoothie)

-Tomatoes

I also added the following supplements and herbs:

-Aloe Vera

-Burdock root tea

-Cardamom

-Yellow dock tea

-Ashwagandha

-Chaga mushrooms

Now, you may be thinking, "Um, Sharon, this seems like a lot to purchase for healing." It was at first, and slowly but surely, I figured out what was working and what supplements seemed to be repeated throughout his books, so I was able to narrow those down considerably. For example, lemon balm, cilantro, dulse, barley grass juice powder, nascent iodine, spirulina, and nettle leaf were mentioned in all of the areas I was dealing with so I basically stuck with those throughout my journey. This is one of those situations where no one can tell you exactly what to do, you have to read and decipher what your own needs are.

If you want to heal, you have to do your homework. You just do.

So, I took this all on over the span of a year and three months, I stumbled, I messed up, I bought the wrong stuff sometimes, but I stuck with it and now I am nearly 100% healed. (Nearly 100% because I am still working on my liver health. I had hurt my liver so bad with my food choices as well as the poison from the spider bites, that it will take a bit longer for my liver to heal, maybe another 6 months, maybe another year but I'm not giving up.) All of the symptoms I mentioned earlier are gone. I feel healthier than I have ever felt in my life, even in my teens and 20's. I am no longer on any synthetic medications for my ADHD, depression, and blood pressure. My doctor has been blown away with what I have accomplished and is now a bit more curious about this guy called 'Medical Medium.' I am living proof that with persistence, study, and the will to heal, ANYTHING can happen.

I have been combing over some videos that might help parents with kids with special needs and this Medical Medium stuff and if you type in 'Medical Medium Autism' or 'Medical Medium ADHD' on YouTube, there are families out there that are living this protocol and seeing results in their kids. It's definitely worth checking out.

I know this chapter, in particular, is a little overwhelming but I felt it was very important to include it so you can see that I personally practice everything that I recommend. I truly believe if you follow the Medical Medium protocol with your child and even yourself, you will see profound results. The first key, in healing your child with special needs, is to get rid of those heavy metals, so, as I said, I prescribe the heavy metal detox smoothie to almost every one of my OT kids. We all have heavy metals inside of us and we will really do ourselves some good by detoxing them.

Again, for further information, please refer to the 'Medical Medium' books on Amazon (also listed in the references) as well as Spanthony's website at www.medicalmedium.com.

Appendix

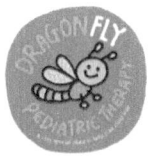

Retained Reflexes Checklist

Child's Name:

_____

Date: _____

*Please check each area that you are seeing in your child consistently.

Fear Paralysis Reflex

___ Seems to have high anxiety overall
___ Poor self-esteem
___ Sleep or eating disorders/issues
___ Above necessary aggression
___ Fear of failure or embarrassment
___ Unexplained phobias

Moro Reflex

___ Carsickness, poor balance, and poor coordination
___ Poor stamina
___ Does not maintain eye contact

___ Sensitive to light
___ Sensitive to sound
___ Allergies
___ Adverse reaction to drugs
___ Hypoglycemic
___ Strongly dislikes change
___ Anxiety or nervousness
___ Mood swings
___ Poor math sense

Babkin Reflex

___ Tendency to clutch fists when unnecessary
___ Hyper-mobility in the fingers
___ Sensitivities in the palms of the hands
___ Difficulties with overall fine-motor
     skills/handwriting/fasteners
___ Moves tongue, lips, or mouth involuntarily
when using hands such as in handwriting
___ Articulation issues
___ Under developed facial expressions

___ Tension in jaw and tooth grinding
___ Regularly chews pencils, fingernails, etc.
___ Has trouble using eating utensils

Rooting Reflex

___ Picky eater
___ Continues to suck thumb at an older age
___ Often drool dribbles from his/her mouth
___ Speech and articulation issues

Palmar Reflex

___ Poor fine motor skills
___ Poor manual dexterity/in-hand manipulation
of objects
___ Poor handwriting

Tonic Labyrinthine Reflex

___ Poor posture
___ Weak muscles
___ Poor balance
___ Unable to cross eyes easily or it hurts to do
so

___ Spatial issues ie: bumps into walls or furniture or stands too close

___ Poor sequencing ie: telling stories, counting, or organizing

___ Poor sense of time, unable to tell time even though he/she should

Spinal Galant

___ Fidgeting

___ Bedwetting

___ Poor concentration or attention

___ Poor memory

___ Very sensitive in several of his/her senses

___ Difficulty reading

Asymmetrical Tonic Neck Reflex

___ Unable to cross eyes or it hurts to do so

___ Eyes jump over words or parts of words, lines, or repeats lines when reading

___ Poor balance

___ Right and left confusion

___ Mixes up d's and b's or other letters or numbers
___ Difficulty skipping or marching
___ Poor handwriting
___ Poor expression of ideas on paper
___ Has not developed hand dominance

Stepping Reflex

___ Toe walks or runs
___ Tight calf muscles
___ Poor balance and muscle control
___ Feet and ankle problems with pain and dysfunction

Heel Reflex

___ Heavy heel walking-walks like a baby elephant through the house
___ Complaints of heel pain
___ Achilles tendonitis-inflammation or complains about Achilles tendon pain
___ Complaints of shin splints

___ Poor core strength/stability
___ Balance problems

Symmetrical Tonic Neck Reflex

___ Poor posture
___ Ape like walk (hunched posture)
___ Poor eye hand coordination
___ Messy eater
___ Unable to cross the eyes or it hurts to do so
___ Slow with copying tasks
___ Poor attention skills

Plantar Reflex

___ Had difficulty learning to walk
___ Runs awkwardly
___ Poor balance
___ Problems playing sports coordinately
___ Has trouble walking in the dark

Sensory Integration Checklist

*Please circle the numbers that apply to your child on a consistent basis

Name: _____ Date:_____

Touch
1. Overreacts to physically painful experiences
2. Underreacts to physically painful experiences
3. Avoids messy activities
4. Craves messy activities
5. Dislikes being touched, especially unexpectedly; is bothers and irritated when crowded and isolates self from others
6. Craves being touched
7. Seeks out physically aggressive contact such as roughhousing, crashing into walls or people
8. Is excessively ticklish
9. Avoids using hands for prolonged periods of time or for examining objects thoroughly

Balance and Movement
1. Has poor balance
2. Has difficulty going up and down stairs or hills
3. Often rocks while sitting in a chair or assumes an upside-down position
4. Often props head in hands while reading or writing
5. Seems fearful in space (e.g. swinging, seesaws, or heights)

6. Is afraid of or avoids vigorous fast-moving activities at the playground (bouncing, swinging, balancing, or spinning)
7. Seems sensitive to movement, getting dizzy, or sea/car sick
8. Prefers fast moving play or seems to never get dizzy with spinning

Coordination
1. Has difficulty with manual skills such as using scissors, crayons, pencils, buttons, and/or handwriting
2. Seems clumsy and accident prone and trips and falls a lot
3. Has difficulty learning new movement activities and/or dislikes trying them
4. Was slow to show a clear hand preference or has not established one
5. Must be reminded to hold the paper while writing
6. Uses extraneous movements during physical activities (e.g. sticks tongue out, moves jaw, or clenches fists)

Muscle Tone
1. Appears stiff and rigid
2. Appears loose and floppy
3. Has poor standing and/or sitting posture
4. Grasps objects too hard or tightly
5. Grasps objects too loosely
6. Tires easily

Hearing
1. Is frightened or irritated by loud noises
2. Is very sensitive to background noise
3. Has difficulty paying attention amid surrounding noises
4. Often shouts or speaks in a loud voice
5. Frequently makes repetitive noises or sounds
6. Fails to follow through on verbal requests
7. Needs directions repeated often
8. Confuses spoken words (e.g. bear/hair)
9. Misses some sounds

Sight
1. Appears sensitive to light, prefers dark or dim lighting
2. Has difficulty discriminating shapes and colors
3. Has difficulty keeping eyes on objects
4. Cannot follow a moving object or line of print well with eyes; loses place
5. Often squints, rubs eyes, gets headaches, or water eyes after reading
6. Becomes excited with a lot of visual stimuli
7. Resists having vision blocked
8. Reverses or confuses numbers, letters, or whole words
9. Has difficultly with written instruction
10. Has difficulty copying from the board or books

Smell

1. Is overly sensitive to certain smells
2. Ignores noxious odors
3. Has difficulty discriminating orders

Attention and Behavior
1. Is restless or fidgety
2. Is impulsive, often jumping up before instructions are given
3. Has difficulty organizing or structuring activities

SENSORY INTEGRATION ACTIVITES

Tactile Integration:
-rub a variety of textures against the skin-child can do this to self
-water play with pitchers and containers in a tub of water
-water painting-painting steps, sidewalk, self, etc. with wet paint brush
-finger painting
-finger drawing-draw on arms or back-guess what shape, letter, etc.
-sand/rice play-objects in sand/rice-find
-feelie box-hole in top of shoe box-hand in-feel and name objects(stereognosis)
-can you find it-in sand or rice with eyes covered
-can you describe it-objects of different sizes, weight, shape, texture, etc.-describe-heavy, soft, etc.-eyes closed
-kneading dough
-handling pets
-swaddle child
-people sandwich-spread the mustard with deep pressure on child's body
-back rubs-deep pressure

-shaving cream drawings
-theraputty/play-dough-rolling into balls-roll the dough
-tactile road-shoes off or crawling with shorts on-rug to mat to bear rug to foam to etc.
-dress up with different texture of clothing
-roll therapy ball on child
Oral Tactile Integration:
-licking stickers and putting in books, on self, poster board, etc.-blowing whistles, kazoos, bubbles thru a straw, chewing gum, Twizzlers

Vestibular Integration:
-hippity hoppity
-roll up child in blanket
-swinging-in all directions
-spinning-sit n' spin
-sliding-different positions
-riding different vehicles-cars, bikes, scooters, etc.
-trampoline
-rocking chair
-walking on an unstable surface
-balancing, walking on see-saw
-sitting on t-stool (increase balance, attention, and posture)
-balancing on teeter-totter
-therapy ball-sitting, on tummy, back, side, etc.

-tummy down-head up activities-reading,
coloring, or watching tv on tummy
-up and down stairs
-summer saults
-running
-v-sitting and doing row boat
-airplane on "mommy's" hands/feet and crash on
 "mommy"
-wheel barrow walking
-donkey kicks

Proprioceptive Integration:
-carrying or pushing heavy loads-pushing a
grocery cart with heavy things inside-carrying a
2 ltr bottle around like a baby or heavy bucket of
water
-pulling-rope tied to a poll
-hanging by arms-monkey bars or chin up bar
-pillow crashing
-hermit crab with shell-bag of rice or beans on
back for shell
-joint compression
-body squeeze-knees against chest-wad child up
and rock back and forth
-bear hugs
-pouring water out of pitchers-different sizes =
 different weights

-ripping paper
-tug of war
-catching large ball or pillow
-arm wrestling
-leap frog
-kicking a paper bag
-hammering
-Theraband stretching
-cleaning mirror
-gum-crunchy foods

Fine-Motor Activities:
-Legos
-blocks
-magnets
-puzzles
-string and lacing
-sorting small objects into egg carton
-cutting, coloring, drawing
-theraputty-squeeze, pound, roll, etc.
-hanging clothes on clothes line
-squeeze a breeze-using an old ketchup or
detergent bottle-squeeze bottle to blow a pieces
of paper across table to score, for example

Motor-Planning Activities:
-obstacle courses-changing body positions-crawling thru tunnels, up and down ramps, balance beams, boards, stepping stones, stairs, ladders, monkey bars, etc.
-jumping from a low surface down onto a mat
-jump to a musical beat
-walking like animals-crab-snake-ostrich (grasp ankles and walk)-duck (squat)-bunny- frog, etc.
-wheel barrow walking/donkey kicks
-Simon Says- ring around the rosy-London bridges
-sports

Bilateral Coordination Activities:
-roll ball with both hands back and forth or use paper towel tubes in each hand to swat back and forth-can use a balloon also
-catch a ball
-with feet still, hit a beach ball with a bat-crossing midline
-bat a balloon
-rolling pin-with theraputty/play dough
-clapping and tapping to music or child follows you
-marble painting
-screwing/unscrewing jars

-jumping rope
-swimming
-bear hunt-using bilateral hands to part grass, swim in the water, claw like a bear, etc.
-tapping two sticks together-rhythm
-Simon says-touching opposite shoulders-crossing midline

Oral-Motor Activities:
-chewy necklaces-licorice necklaces, cheerios necklaces, tubing
-drink applesauce through a straw
-blow cotton balls or any light weight ball across the table with or without a straw for a "soccer" game or race
-blow up under a tissue trying to keep it afloat
-blow up a balloon and let it go-try to catch it
-chewing gum-blow bubble-measure to see whose is bigger
-making emotional/funny faces in the mirror
-kiss the mirror or paper with lipstick on and then draw figures out of the lipstick kiss marks-butterfly

Visual Skill Activities:
-flashlight tag-2 flashlights-you shine yours to a part of a darkened room-child hand to look for your flashlight and point his onto your spot
-mazes-dot to dot
-drawing shapes and letter into finger paint, shaving cream, etc.
-rubber band boards-copying patterns
-peg board designs
-jigsaw puzzles, building blocks
-find all of the o's, t's, p's in the paragraph in the newspaper or magazine
-trails
-word search

Alerting Activities:
-crunching foods
-taking a shower
-bouncing on a therapy ball
-jumping up and down on a trampoline

Organizing Activities:
-chewing granola bars, fruit bars, licorice, or/and gum
 -hanging by hands from monkey bars or chin-up bar

-pushing or pulling heavy loads
-any upside-down position

<u>Calming Activities:</u>
-sucking a pacifier, hard candy(sucking), frozen fruit bars, or spoonful of peanut butter
-pushing against a wall with hands, shoulders, back, butt, and head
-rocking, swaying, or swinging slowly back and forth
-cuddling-back rubs
-taking a bath

Websites I Recommend:

1. www.autismspeaks.org- Autism Speaks provides a comprehensive resource guide for all 50 states. It also has a great list of apps that parents will find very useful.

2. www.autism.healingthresholds.com- Healing Thresholds provides information on the many different therapy treatments for children with autism.

3. www.autismbeacon.com- Autism Beacon provides articles on autism including sensitive subjects such as sexuality and bullying.

4. www.autism-society.org- The Autism Society gives helpful resources for

parents as well as professionals as well as updates on the latest news and press releases.

5. www.autism.com- The Autism Research Institute focuses on researching the causes of autism as well as treatments.

6. www.disabilityscoop.com- This website provides an e-mail newsletter on the most current updates on developmental disabilities.

7. www.autismweb.com- AutismWeb provides insights on different teaching techniques for autism. It also provides a forum for parents.

8. www.autismhwy.com- Autism Highway provides a list of autism related events and specialists.

9. https://pottygenius.com/potty-training-a-child-with-autism-using-aba/- A great resource for helping potty train your child using ABA methods.

10. www.additudemag.com- An excellent resource for information on ADD/ADHD for both children and adults.

11. www.adhdchildhood.com- A great website for resources and information about ADD/ADHD.

12. www.chadd.org- Another great website for resources and information about ADD/ADHD.

13. There are a ton more but these are the ones that I find myself visiting and recommending the most. There are

also a ton of blogs about parenting a child with special needs. Some of the top ADHD blogs can be found here: www.healthline.com/health/adhd/best-blogs-of-the-year#1 Some of the top autism blogs can be found here: www.healthline.com/health/autism/best-blogs-of-the-year#1

14. www.dragonflypediatricot.com- This is my own website and I have it chalk full of helpful information from apps that I recommend to therapy toys that I use and recommend. There are also links to my Pinterest site as well as my Facebook site where I also post helpful information and tips. When I have time, I also blog on my website.

Last but not least, the recipe for my infamous 'Shumalings!'

-Using an 8 oz cup of your choice, fill crushed ice all the way to the top

-Pour in 2 ounces of your choice of vodka

-Pour in 3 ounces of Malibu

-Add a splash of lemon and a splash of lime

-Then fill the rest of the cup up with cranberry juice

-Mix well and enjoy!

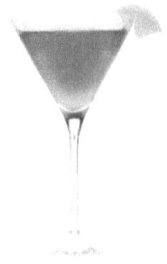

References

1. Blakeslee, Sandra and Matthew. 'The Mind Has A Body of Its Own.' New York. Random House, Inc., 2007.
2. Gerber M.D., Richard. 'Vibrational Medicine.' Rochester, VT. Bear and Company, 2001.
3. Bealle, Morris Allison. 'The Drug Story.' Washington, D.C. Columbia Publishing Company, 1949.
4. Bleecker, LAC, MSOM, Deborah. 'Acupuncture Points Handbook.' Draycott Publishing, 2017.
5. Hayes, Tim. 'The Power of Horses to Heal.' New York. St. Martin's Press, 2016.
6. Blomberg, M.D., Harald with Dempsey, Moira. 'Movements That Heal...' Australia. Beyond the Sea Squirt, 2011.
7. Northrup, M.D., Christiane. 'The Subtle Body' Boulder, CO. Sounds True, Inc., 2009.

8. Brandes, MEd, Bonnie L. 'The Symphony of Reflexes.' North Charleston, NC. CreateSpace Independent Publishing Platform, 2015.
9. 'Essential Oils.' Berkley, CA. Althea Press, 2015.
10. Goddard, Sally. 'Reflexes, Learning, and Behavior.' Eugene, OR, 2002.
11. Walbarger, M.S., Julia. 'The Wilbarger Protocol.'
Retrieved from www.nationalautismsource.com.
12. Gallaway, OD, Michael. 'Vision and Learning.'
Retrieved from www.drgallaway.com.
13. Freedman, Cindy and Tisser, Ailene. 'The Benefitsvof Aquatic Therapy for Special Needs Children.' Retrieved from www.theaquatictherapist.com.
14. Patino, Erica. 'Biofeedback: What It Is and How It Works.'
15. Muse: The Brain Sensing Headband information and picture were used with permission from the Gaiam Company.

16. HeartMath.com. The Inner Balance
    information
    and picture was used with permission from
    HeartMath.
17. Retained Neonatal Reflexes. 'Reflexes
    Explained.'
    Retrieved from
    www.retainedneonatalreflexes.com.au.
18. Facebook quote. 'What is Vibrational
    Frequency?'
    fb.com/crystalhealingconnection.
19. Piper-Terry, M.S., Marcella. 'Vaccines Do
    Not Cause Autism.' Retrieved from
    www.vaxtruth.org.
20. Paul, Kathi. Happy Trails Therapeutic
    Riding Center. Retrieved from
    www.happytrailstrc.org.
21. Plant Therapy. Plant Therapy gave
permission to appear in this book as well and the
use of their timeline picture. Retrieved from
    www.planttherapy.com.
21. Frick, Sheila. Therapeutic Listening.
    Retrieved
    from www.vitalsounds.com.

22. Interactive Metronome Therapy. Retrieved from
www.interactivemetronome.com.

24. Brain Beat. Retrieved from
www.brainbeat.com.

25. PATH. Retrieved from
https://www.pathintl.org.

26. American Hippotherapy Association, Inc.
Retrieved from
www.americanhippotherapyassociation.org.

27. Amor, Jaime. Cosmic Kids Yoga. Retrieved
from
https://training.cosmickids.com.

28. Kranowitz, M.A., Carol Stock. 'The Out of
Sync
Child.' USA. Penguin Publishing Group,
1998.

29. Kranowitz, M.A., Carol Stock. 'The Out of
Sync
Child Has Fun.' Tarcher Perigee, 2006.

30. Health Science Academy. 'Nutritional
Therapist
Certification. Retrieved from

https://courses.thehealthsciencesacademy.org.

31. Batterson, Mark. 'Draw the Circle.' Austin, TX.

    Fedd and Company, Inc., 2012.
32. Stein, Ph.D., Steven J., Book, M.D., 'The EQ Edge.' Ontario. Multi-Health Systems, Inc., 2011.
33. Interactive Metronome Therapy. Retrieved from

    www.interactivemetrone.com.
34. Eye Can Learn. Retrieved from

    www.eyecanlearn.com.
35. Auditory Transduction. Retrieved from

    https://youtu.be/PeTriGTENoc.
36. Oetter, Patricia. Richter, Eileen. Frick, Sheila M.

    'M.O.R.E.' PDP Press, 1993.
37. William, Anthony. 'Medical Medium.' Hay House, Inc., 2015.
38. William, Anthony. 'Medical Medium Liver Rescue.' Hay House, Inc., 2018.
39. William, Anthony. 'Medical Medium Life-Changing Foods.' Hay House, Inc., 2016.
40. William, Anthony. 'Medical Medium Thyroid Healing.' Hay House, Inc., 2016.
41. William, Anthony. 'Medical Medium Celery Juice.' Hay House, Inc., 2019.

42. Whitten, Ari. 'The Ultimate Guide to Red Light Therapy.' Archangel Ink, 2018.

43. The Canadian Association for Music Therapy.
    'What is Music Therapy.' May 1994.

44. Autism Speaks. 'What is Applied Behavior Analysis?' www.autismspeaks.org.

45. Psychology Today. 'Parent-Child Interaction Therapy (PCIT).' 2019.

46. Silver Linings Neurodevelopment website at www.silverliningsclinic.com.

47. Rhythmic Movement Training International.
    'What is Rhythmic Movement?' www.rhythmicmovement.org.

48. Association for Play Therapy. 'What is Play Therapy?' www.a4pt.org.

49. Top 10 Autism Websites Recommended by Parents. Eden II Programs. 2019

50. God. 'The Bible.' Heaven. The Word. Eternity.

www.ingramcontent.com/pod-product-compliance
Lightning Source LLC
Chambersburg PA
CBHW030608220526
45463CB00004B/1221